Amazing Love Diet

Dorothy D Stover

USA

I dedicate this book to the women in my life, especially my Mother. You have shown me real beauty, and what it means to love yourself for who you really are.

Foreword

This is the second edition of Amazing Love Diet. I pulled the first edition off the shelves due to the sexual content and my amazing spelling and grammatical errors. (Can you believe it? I even spelled grammar wrong!)

Obviously spelling is not my forte. I think of myself as an ideas girl. I am usually 'in my head,' thinking about whatever is going on up there. I love to write, which is why that's what I do. Am I any good at it? Perhaps. Is the content in this book information that I happen to be the only one who understands, or knows? No. This book is a compilation of what I have learned in (what some consider) my few, short years on this planet. I am still learning and discovering. I am an observer, and I have a great memory for events. This has enabled me to tell you what I know. At least, a small portion of what I have learned. A girl has to save some secrets for herself!

When I first set out to write this book I was excited and thrilled. I thought about writing this book for many years before I ever set my fingers to the keyboard. As time went on and I was engrossed in writing, I realized how much of myself I was actually putting into this book. The thought that people would know so much about me was, and is, so scary. That was the primary reason for my taking so long to complete the first edition, and why it has taken me so long to complete this second edition. It's as if I am walking down the street completely naked and exposed. There are certainly moments when I love being in my invisible bikini and strutting my stuff like the proud lioness that I am. Then there are those frightening moments when I realize I am the only one without cover, and I begin to rethink my courage to stand apart from the crowd.

Amazing Love Diet

Once I started this book there was no other option but to finish. I have completed this journey of writing Amazing Love Diet. I am proud of myself for taking a risk and putting myself out there. I hope you enjoy this glimpse into my world. I hope you are entertained, and perhaps learn something you didn't know before. I hope that you are inspired. Inspired to love. Inspired to live life to the fullest. Inspired to branch out and take your own risks in life. The reward could be great. You'll only know if you try. Thank you so much for your support, and as always Much Love to You.

PS. Sorry to anyone who was really looking forward to the Sexercises. I plan on releasing that information in more detail in a future publication.

The Beginning - My Story

"All our knowledge has its origins in our perceptions."
-Leonardo da Vinci

Within this book you will find the secrets to a beautiful body. Achieving this is easier than you might think. I have put in years of research, time and experience through my travels to find the story of how love can transform your body and your mind. I am living proof that the effort one puts into love can yield a greater reward.

For you to truly understand this book, you need to know where I am coming from. I have a few stories about how I became me! My first story will be about my body and mind. The second is a story about love. The third story is a mystery! (This trifecta ultimately revealed me to ME!) This is the foundation. Later in the book, I will share with you my secrets to love and achieving a beautiful body. Love, and what we put in our bodies, plays a major role in achieving this.

My Body and Mind

There are many different aspects to my body. I am tall. I am never the same weight two days in a row. I wear glasses. I have wavy, unruly hair. I have small feet. I am awkward. I have an hourglass figure. I have a pointy nose. I have small hands. I have hazel eyes. I have an "innie" for a bellybutton. My voice resembles that of a five year old. I am a bad speller. I love to eat. I love to drink Champagne. My grammar is wretched. I can't do a cartwheel. Open water calms me down. I am obsessive. I am lazy. I am energetic. (I am contradictory!) I have long legs. I am territorial. I can be weird. I talk too much. I am happy. I love.

I didn't know anything was wrong with me until I started grade school. Children have a spectacular way of singling someone out. First of all, I was smaller in stature than the other kids and extremely thin. I wore glasses and marched (frenziedly) to a different drummer. This combination isn't a good one for being popular. It was difficult even getting by without someone taking the time to notice me in a negative light. This all added up to many days coming home crying to my Mother who always knew exactly what to say to make me feel better. "You tell those kids that if they don't leave you alone, I'm going to come down there and hang them up by their toes."

My mother is a powerhouse standing at about 5' 2" with flaming red hair. She may be little in size but you would never want to mess around with her, or make my mother angry. You would soon come to the realization that doing so was a bad idea. So, backed with my mother's strong spirit, I held my head higher and started to fight my own battles. Sometimes with my fists, sometimes with words. Soon children in grade school did stop picking on me, but they would eventually pick on someone else. In turn, I found myself fighting for others who, like me, were afraid to speak up, or defend themselves against the terrifying eight year olds.

As time went on I became more awkward and my height shot up to make me one of the tallest in the class. This really didn't help my case as I was still super-thin and had my bottle cap glasses. Children came up with very clever names like "Spider Dot" or "Dotty-long-legs." My mother gave me solid, wonderful, wise advise. She would say to me, "Just ignore them. Nothing makes someone angrier than when you ignore them." I found this statement to be nonsensical at the time. I wanted to take my abnormally small hands and ring their little necks. I thought this would be the best way to shut them up. Eventually, after much consideration, I took my mother's advice and just ignored the kids. I learned to develop a thick skin where name-calling was concerned.

Our growing-up years lay the foundation for who we are, and who we will become. Our parents can only do their best and what they consider is right for their children.

Society can also play a major role in how we act and feel about ourselves. It's sad, but it's the truth. We all have short comings that people are more than happy to expose and profit over, all while overlooking their own. Every event, every experience, every person who touches our lives, even the ones that seem insignificant at the time, all shape who we are.

When I was 19 years old, I became very sick. I was taking roughly 23 supplements daily and was only allowed to eat certain foods. The main food items I had to cut out were dairy, wheat, yeast and gluten. At the time there weren't as many healthy food choices on the shelves in the grocery that met my requirements. Even at health food stores it was hard to find food that met all of my needs. Sure, there were some items available, but not the selection that we know today. Now you may walk into any common grocery store and find something that will conform to most dietary restrictions, and it will taste good. Almost like the real thing! Almost.

The lowest point in my food life was right after I was diagnosed. My mother took me to the grocery store to gather all my new "eats." Moms in general know how to make everything better, and my mother in particular has quite the talent for it. She made me feel special and cared for. Unfortunately, that all disappeared when I was sitting in my dorm room craving a grilled cheese sandwich, one of my favorite comfort foods. I wasn't going to let this "bump in the road" stop me from enjoying life, and I was determined to make my own grilled cheese sandwich.

I took out my wheat free, yeast free, gluten free, (taste free) cardboard bread and added my "plastic-looking" rice cheese to the center of the two slices. I took out my toaster oven. (Now, I know you're not supposed to have a toaster oven in your dorm room. I had special permission because of my circumstances.) I placed my little makeshift grilled cheese in the toaster oven. I continued to watch my grilled cheese with anticipation. I was so excited for it to be done, and couldn't wait to sink my teeth into something yummy and gooey. As I stared through the glass at my sandwich, my smile started to turn upside down. I watched as the edges of the bread turned upwards away from the rice "plastic-looking" cheese. Then the buzzer went off. With a positive attitude and a grumbling stomach I took out my little sandwich and had my first bite. This was followed by tears streaming down my face. I sat in my dorm room crying and couldn't stop crying and continued to eat my grilled cheese. To my surprise and disappointment my sandwich didn't have any of the yummy, comforting gooeyness that I was craving. Instead, this grilled cheese tasted just like it looked: two pieces of cardboard with a slice of plastic in the middle. That was my lowest moment in my food life. (I would learn a valuable lesson that day: never cry while you're eating.)

Now, I had to change my diet to save my life and to get better. Eventually, I did get my health back and once I was healed, I was able to add certain foods back into my diet. You may not be in such a predicament, but still your life and food situation is just as critical as mine was. You need to get yourself to the healthy point, and then you can start adding more foods into your diet. Our bodies are always in need of balance.

On to my second story about Love.

Love

Growing up, I was obsessed with love and finding my soul mate. I was a true romantic. As a child, all I wanted to do was get married to someone who I loved madly, and who loved me back in the same way. We would make a family together! For many years I carried around a tiny toy baby. I loved this baby more than anything and truly believed I was this toy baby's mother.

Over time, my excessive love for this baby would result in a weakening of the doll's fabric "skin." A tear in a leg, an arm, or her torso would appear, here or there, and would have to be duct-taped. Within a few years the baby had a duct-tape diaper and body suit. The painted on eyes started to fade and my baby looked more like a grey ball of duck tape than the cute snuggly baby that it once had been. That is a part of love, isn't it? The original thing we started off with changes shape, becoming something completely different, almost to the point of being unrecognizable. The only thing that recognizes it is your heart's eye. Your heart has vision better than 20/20.

My one was goal in life at a very early age was to fall in love. When I learned what people did with each other when they were in love (sex), well, this just fueled my drive for love and my search for my soul mate. I had the scenario all planned in my head. I would lose my virginity to the person I was going to be with for the rest of my life. We would have a beautiful night of sweet kisses, caressing each other's bodies, and intense, soulful eye contact. This was my dream and I would wait until the day I found this special person. We would give ourselves, our whole selves, to each other. It was a sweet dream, one I held onto, even to this day.

The years passed, my body and I changed, but I never abandoned my ultimate goal. Of course, I felt pressure in middle school and high school to find someone to lose my virginity to. My friends all had boyfriends. And me? Well, it was a rarity for any boy to look at me since I towered over most of them and resembled a two-by-four board with Coke-bottle glasses and had braces to boot. I still put pressure on myself, thinking, he's just around the corner. You just have to wait a little bit longer.

As time went on I thought if I was going to find someone, I'd better look more like my friends. They all had shapely bodies and wore more revealing clothing. I come from a very strict Catholic family with conservative parents. At least where fashion was concerned. Wearing a skirt, shorts or a shirt that was too short was forbidden. I remember coming down all dressed for school one morning, and started making my breakfast. I reached up to the top cabinet for my favorite cereal – Cinnamon Toast Crunch. My Mother yelped, "Is that your belly? Go change your shirt." My shirt was (maybe) showing an inch of my skin while my hands were above my head. When my parents would stop me, abruptly, from leaving the house in whatever get up I may have been wearing, all I could think about was, "I'll never find a boyfriend. And I'll never have sex." I would later go on to find out it truly doesn't matter what someone may look like or what someone may wear. If you want sex, more than likely someone will be ready and willing to oblige you. I have also discovered that there is someone for everyone. If you have a big nose, I bet there is someone out there who is going to think your nose is the sexiest nose on the planet. Best advice: Just be who you are, someone will fall in love with the genuine you.

Fashion-wise growing up, I was a bit of a dud. My parents had less than no interest in buying me clothes that were fashionable, like the other girls my age. They didn't want me dressing too "mature" for my age, and with good reason.   There are some creepy, disturbed people in this world who prey upon young girls.

So, afflicted with conservative parents, a body that looked like a very long stick with glasses, and no fashion sense, in my own eyes I was doomed to never finding my soul mate. It was so rare that any guy, besides those over 40, would find me attractive. Soon, I found myself not believing the guy if he did like me.

I once read a book that said that before we come on to this earth we choose our families. Evidently, before we get here, somehow we know what we have to work on during our lifetime, and we know how long we will stay on this earth. I would say I am starting to agree with this statement. I have always believed we know what we're supposed to be when we grown up at a very young age. We know what impact we are going to make on the world by the time we're five. At least in my opinion we do. Perhaps our parents have a different vision for us than the one we have. This, too, is part of what will shape and mold who you become. For the most part, we already "know" what we are going to be, we just don't know the details of the journey.

As a child, I didn't know what "being in love" was, but I knew that was for me! I wanted to meet my soul mate and grow old together. When I graduated from high school my Mother gave me a present. It was some type of time capsule. It was just a box made out of cardboard that she found at some store like Borders or Barnes and Noble. I remember her presenting this gift to me. The "capsule" was actually a shiny, blue, rectangular box with a painted-on yellow ribbon across the front. I opened up the box like a box of Russell Stover chocolates to find multiple questionnaires with matching envelopes. I was supposed to hand each questionnaire to a friend or family member to fill out. I also had my own questionnaire to fill out. Once all the questionnaires were completed each person would seal their envelope and place it in the box. I would have to wait 10 years before being able to open each letter. Talk about anticipation!

Throughout those 10 years of waiting, I remember wondering what my family and friends would write about me. How did they see my future? Will I be a completely different person in 10 years, or will I be the same? Will everything that I want come true? Ten years did eventually pass. One day, out of the blue, I came upon the blue time capsule box. I was extremely nervous and apprehensive about what I was going to find inside. I opened each envelope with excitement and enthusiasm. It felt like

Christmas and each letter was a small gift for me to unwrap! Much to my surprise, the life that people thought I would be living was quite different than the reality. It was as different as the world I had thought for myself. My family, friends and I all thought that by age 28 or 29, I would be married with a family!

Little did I know back then, but it's a long road from where you think you should be and where you are. I have experienced more pain than I would want my worst enemy to go through. Still, with all the heartache and pain, I believe in love. I still believe in the good. I still hope. I have found the good through love of myself, travel, and love of others. Let me share with you what I've learned thus far on my journey in life. I believe the love of ourselves is the greatest treasure we will ever behold.

The Journey to Love

"And think not you can direct the course of love, for love, if it finds you worthy, directs your course."
-Khalil Gibran

"To thine own self be true." I believe Shakespeare meant this line to mean, "Take care of yourself first." I also believe you shouldn't take this as an excuse to be selfish. Certainly though, you must secure your own oxygen mask before helping others secure theirs. What good are you to others if you are not 100%? This is a lesson I have learned over and over again. Take care of yourself, before taking care of others. The journey to Love is a journey to loving yourself. Loving yourself, in turn, allows you to have the body and the life that you need. (Notice how I didn't say want?) What we want, may not be and most likely is not, what we need. I would love to be 5'2" and 110 pounds. Guess what? That will never happen and I've accepted it. Love yourself for your unique self, eat well, and love every moment, even if you have pain in your heart.

I have often felt that life is beautiful. Almost perfect, the way things seem to work out. Even in my darkest moments I've tried to find the good. Eventually the good always finds a way back into my life. Those dark moments are the real moments in our lives that truly shape the person who we are and who we will become. It's those moments when we are staring at fear and pain that really make life worth living. If every day were perfect, you wouldn't actually know what perfect was. If you never had a bad day, you would never know what a good day feels like. So, when you do experience the bad in life, remember it. Learn from it. Heal from it, knowing that good is around the corner, waiting silently for you. I would care to wager, that once you've experience the bad, you hold on that much tighter to the good in life. Maybe even treasure it just a little more than when you did in your past. I know I have and do.

When I have bad days, weeks, months or even years, it gives me comfort to know that somewhere in my future there will be good again. The journey to love is rough terrain. There are ups and downs. There will be moments when you don't believe you are worth it and then there will be moments when you know you are.

In my experience, and what I have observed in my few years on this planet, is most people go through some sort of trauma. This acts as a trigger. This trigger may set you off on an unhealthy path. Maybe even a destructive path. This is just a mere distraction if you break down the trigger. Once you have discovered what your particular trigger is that set you on an unhealthy path, you will be empowered to change what you need to change to chart your course on to the smoother road to love.

How to discover your trigger:

For me, I tried to diligently keep track of how I feel, what I do when something upsets me. What I discovered was, when I am upset or in need of comfort I tend to turn to food. I have noticed that when I am unhappy, even if I am eating fairly well, I still gain weight. When I am happy in my life, somehow pounds just fall off and stay off. So, my greatest health secret is to be happy with myself and love myself...But that you already know.

To discover what may set you off on the wrong path listen to what happens to your mind, your body, and your spirit when something upsets you. What do you remember? Write everything down, even if it seems small and insignificant. It's sometimes the little things in our everyday that can make us upset and create a toxin in our system.

I know for me when a romantic relationship ends, it triggers a lot of my bad habits. I won't eat right. I won't take walks or be active in any way. I hit rock bottom every-time, until I am able to recognize that this is one of my triggers. Sure, I still grab a bag of BBQ chips and a pint of Ben and Jerry's Half Baked but I don't hate myself for it. I recognize that it's a temporary fix. Then I move on and do the work to move on from the relationship and get myself back to 100% both in body, mind and spirit.

I have found in my past that even when I was in a relationship I was truly single. So I learned to love myself. If I didn't love who I was then how could someone love me if I didn't love myself? I think this is simple logic, just not as simple to accomplish. I have often found myself comparing my mind and body to others. When I should accept myself for who I am, all of my talents and all of my beauties.

Here is a Self-Love Exercise, Beautiful Body, which I have taught others. This exercise will help you to fall in love with your own body. This may take time and repetitive repetitions to gain the full benefits. Anything worth achieving does require effort and work on each individual.

I suggest you start off by looking at your naked body in the mirror. Be your best friend. Best friends will always tell you that you look beautiful and bring your spirits up. So what would your friends say to you? Start off by pointing out the positive in yourself. What is your favorite feature? Maybe it's your eyes, butt, and legs or maybe it's your chest, arms and feet. Whatever the case may be, it's all you and you should enjoy it. No one else on this planet is put together quite like you, and that's something to be proud of.

Over time, the effort you made in appreciating yourself, you will find that you are happier with you and your body. You will be amazed what a happier you will do for your spirit and your health. You may even find yourself accepting those dimples on your tummy or cellulite on your thighs. Start today, take off all your clothes and bask in the glory of you and your body.

THE AMAZING LOVE DIET IS BORN

"Take care of your body. It's the only place you have to live."

- Jim Rohn

Family Girl

I am very close to my family. They are my best friends and biggest supporters. I come from a large, loud family, sort of like the one in My Big Fat Greek Wedding. There are always a dozen simultaneous conversations going on, everyone talking to the point you can hardly hear. And, there is always amazing food! I would much rather stay home and watch a movie with my family and eat and eat and eat than to go out "drinking until I can't see any more!"

I just love my family. We laugh all the time, we fight like crazy people, and we always have something delicious for dinner and dessert. I am one of six children. I have two older brothers who would steal the food off my fork. I have an older sister who showed me "the ropes," and told me what to do. I have two younger sisters who I bossed around and tried to make my personal "slaves." Growing up in a big family you gain an enhanced appreciation for food, especially in sufficient quantities. My friends found it incredible how fast I could eat and how I didn't say a word during a meal. The reason for this was, with six kids (and two big older brothers) if you didn't eat fast, you didn't eat. The food was so good and there were plenty of mouths that wanted to eat it. If I wanted seconds, and didn't want my big brothers to eat the food right off my fork, I had to move quickly. So, my food obsession started with my family and my mother's cooking. There is nothing like my mother's cooking. Dessert, for sure, is her specialty and I couldn't get enough.

My experience filling a void with food was something I discovered was while I was going to school in

Florida. I was happy living there. I had great friends, I loved my school, and it was sunny almost all of the time. Coming from the Northeast, that sunny weather was a blessing. I was used to freezing winters, a rainy spring, sticky summers and a grey fall. The problem with Florida was, I discovered, I missed my family. I stuffed my mouth with food. I wasn't listening to my body and its dietary needs. I wasn't eating because I was hungry, and I wasn't eating food that was good for me, I was eating because I missed my family. I gained about 30 pounds of "missing." No one really noticed because I am 5'10" so I was able to hide it well. I went on eating like this for quite some time, just to comfort myself and to attempt to fill the void. Well, at least I thought I did. I once asked my one of my brothers if he could tell I gained weight. His reply, "A little." I had developed this unhappy food habit, and my quality of life went down. I also started seeing a real jerk of a guy who didn't care about my needs, just his own. Funny when you're not 100% you attract others who are not 100%. For a half a year, I wallowed in this mess. Then, BOOM! I finally ended it with the guy and decided I was going to look and feel amazing!

I first started with a list of what I wanted and formed my goals were. I wanted a tip-top shape of a peach, aka my vagina. I wanted my head of hair to grow faster and stronger. I wanted my skin to glow. I researched and found the foods that would facilitate these results. That list of helpful food was all I ate during this time of my recreating myself. I also wasn't dating anyone at this time and kept to my normal routine of pleasuring myself. Honestly, sometimes it isn't worth the trouble of being in a relationship. Especially, if your partner is selfish in bed and in life. What is the point of being with them? So you don't feel alone? You're alone, trust me. You just have someone around to remind you of how alone you are. Once I realized this and kept to the diet, I found that within a month or two I had completely changed my body. My skin, hair, and peach were glowing! (And, I had six-pack abs.) I lost 25 pounds in just a few short months and kept it off.

The birth of the Amazing Love Diet! With more research, I found you can eat for great sex. This great sex doesn't have to be with a partner. I know this because I'm the type of girl who wants a monogamous relationship. I haven't had many partners for fear of what my Mother had always told me: "You will become attached to every person you sleep with." This statement has always scared "the real" into me. Much like what you might say to a child when they've swallowed their chewing gum, "Don't swallow that gum. It will stay in your belly forever!" With this fear of inappropriate attachments, I became the type of girl who could please herself sexually. Practice makes perfect, or so I've heard.

I wasn't going to sleep with just anyone. Even now, as then, there are rigid pre-qualifications: I have to be in love with him, or have a crazy-strong physical attraction to that person. Either one is not easy for me. (Probably why I found myself flying solo!) I have to know he's in it for the long haul, and can handle me. I'm a lot to handle behind closed doors, and not for the faint of heart. My best 48 hours with a guy, we didn't eat any food whatsoever, and I think we got a total of two hours of sleep. When we did come up for air, we ordered take out. So you can see, you have to keep up! I'm the Energizer Bunny. Sometimes sex is "food" for me, and sometimes food is "sex for me." I'm in a constant balancing act.

When I was 12 years old, I read an article on exercise and orgasms, and how they coincide. The article listed 30 different forms of exercise. Some examples: Yoga, Pilates, Running, Walking, Horse Back Riding, Swimming, etc. Along with this helpful list was a poll asking 100 women from each different exercise group about certain aspects of their lifestyle, concentrating on fitness, health and their sex lives. The data was gathered and quantified. The article then listed each exercise along with the percentage of women who experienced frequent orgasms within each grouping. The bottom of this list was running or jogging. Only 23% of women who ran for exercise had frequent orgasms. The top of the list was Pilates, rating at 99% of women having frequent orgasms. I bought a Pilates DVD the very next day.

I should disclose (and my parents will be relieved to learn) that I was not sexually active at 12 years old. Far, far from it. I have had an obsession with sex all my life, even before I really knew what the birds and the bees were. I have always been a fervent reader, gleaning as much information as possible on the subject. You may consider this your gain, as I will pass on my knowledge to you! (Well, as much knowledge as someone can gain at my age and experience.)

As you may have guessed, I am obsessed with sex, always have been, and always will be. I wanted to be sure that when the day finally came for me to be "a woman," I was going to be the best in bed. So, I would kiss every wall in my house, or practice on my hand with the hope that, one day, it would be a real honest-to-goodness tall, dark and handsome man or woman. I was open to all possibilities. The kissing obsessions soon lead to everything to do with sex. I was a sponge, taking all this information in. Now that I am older, I have been able to put my studying into use. In bed I am what they call a "pleaser." I want to make sure my partner is satisfied. I learn what they like, what they really like, and I do it. For me, my pleasure comes from pleasing someone else. I also know how to please myself. I've been practicing since I was about three or four years old. Back then, I didn't know what I was doing, but it felt great. I realized when I got older what was going on. I'll get into that later, because it's important to know how to please yourself.

Amazing Love Diet

To repeat, food and sex have always been my passions. I believe, because I was always so obsessed with sex and my body, it has given me an advantage sexually. When I finally learned to read, I would gather all the information I could on sex. My primary goal was to be the best in bed for my future spouse. Naturally, all this information wouldn't be in play until many, many years down the road, but I wanted to be ready for it, nevertheless!

In my years on this planet, I have found that health and a beautiful body begin within your mind. When you really want something, you are willing to invest whatever it takes to acquire your desire. Whether it be shopping for just the right dress for an up-coming party, or finding the perfect birthday present for that special someone. The desire and the want all start in your mind. The compulsion to get that "perfect something" all starts within you.

When I was a little girl, I told my mother at our dinner table that the way to get a boy to love you was to bat your eyelashes. She just smiled and said, "Oh! Is that how it's done?" I have always had an obsession with love. In some circles they would call it "a passion". For me, it truly was.

Being in love is one of the most amazing feelings you can ever experience. I had a great love, and let me tell you, he could do no wrong in my eyes. Every day I would run to that door to greet the man I couldn't stand to be without. I was much like a puppy. He could have come home and said, "Well it's done. I've killed everyone, and I mean everyone! We are the only two people left." In my sick way, I would have thought, How romantic. I have the best guy ever! Granted, that is an amazing love, but amazingly messed up. Happily, that kind of "love" has faded, and the journey continues.

Amazing Love Diet

For as long as I can remember, my Mother has given me self-help books. They are mainly in regard to love and relationships. It started off with the best seller, Are you there God? It's Me, Margaret. This original self-help book relates a young girl's trials of loving her new body and God. After this little gem, my Mother was on a roll, gifting me with only the crème de la crème of self help books. Books like, He's Just Not That into You, and Steve Harvey's book, Act like a Lady, Think like a Man. Recently, I came to the edge when she handed me her latest find, How to Know If He's Going to Marry You In 30 Days or Less. Now, all things being considered, I'm a lucky girl. I've had a few marriage proposals, some of them serious, some of them not. I'm a girl who loves love and would someday like to have a spouse and a few ankle biters of my own. I believe I would thrive as a wife and mother. It could very well be my calling in life.

I have always been obsessed with finding the right partner to spend the rest of my life with. My Mother and I have a strong bond, and certainly this obsession has played a role in our bond. Over the years, I've had some bad luck in the love department, but I've had some magical moments, too. Falling in love is a beautiful thing. Falling out of love is a process we all have to go through to grow. "Grow with love," as they say.

There was one guy I really thought was going to make my dreams a reality. Except the reality was, I wasn't ready to get married! I had many items on my "Things to Do Before 'I Do' " list. This was a considerably long list, consisting of all my wants and desires. I wanted to travel by myself. I wanted to crash a wedding. I wanted a small career success, and many, many more fun things I just couldn't do if I were married. My desire to be in a healthy, happy marriage notwithstanding, I wasn't quite ready to be in wedded bliss, especially with this list looming over me. Recently I realized that I don't have anything left to do on my list! Maybe, just maybe, I'm ready now that I've completed all the "To Do's?"

My mother has seen me struggle over the years within my romantic relationships, as well as with my weight. She is always trying to help me find my way. This is what makes her a great mother. She wants only the best for me. That was the reason she was constantly handing me the self-help books. It was just another way of trying to help me find my way. I understand where my mother was coming from. It was from a place of love. She only wanted me to be happy. She's seen my heart get broken, but she also wants grand-babies before she's in diapers herself. She knows I've always wanted children, and that playing 'house' was my favorite game as a little girl.

What is this need to see the ones we love paired off, and married? My older sister married when she was twenty-five years old. I was twenty-three at the time. My grandmother said to me the week of the wedding, right after I had broken up with my boyfriend, "Don't worry dear. Twenty-three isn't considered an old maid anymore." I was in shock. Happily, she followed up her comment with, "You're beautiful. You'll have no trouble finding a husband." Thanks, Granny! (I think?)

With so many "self-help" books out there I wanted to write something that was really about "helping you." I love the term, "self -help book." This terminology openly states and affirms that all you need is your self. You are the only person who can help yourself. Sure, others can inspire you and guide you on your path, but when it comes down to the work, you are the only person for the job. You don't need to be anything more than who you are. My goal is for women to feel beautiful about themselves, and to have great sex! That's all I want for them. This sex can be by yourself, or with a partner. I don't want you to count calories, or to worry about if you eat this or that, or berating yourself if you fall off the wagon. Those activities only bring you down. Truthfully, that is no way to live and enjoy life. To me, that is what I live for. I want to enjoy this life. Eat the foods I want, kiss the people I want and bask in how glorious it all was, and is. There are only a few people in this world who are truly happy counting calories. Doctors have a term for those people so afflicted: they are "suffering from" an eating disorder. No offense, but it's true. I am my happiest when I'm around friends and family, enjoying my favorite foods, laughing, and having a glass of very good wine. To me, that's what is worth living for (...and of course great sex!)

The key to a great sex life is confidence and knowing your body. Confidence comes from feeling good about yourself. With this way of life, you will feel better about yourself. You will, in turn, learn things about your body you never knew, or didn't want to admit. You might end up losing 10, 20, 30, or more pounds, but that is not the end goal. That is a bonus. The end goal is to feel beautiful and to have a great time with or without someone behind closed doors. And come on; let's face it that would mean a happy life, even if you couldn't lose those last few pounds.

I will tell you this: our bodies were made for sex. In fact we are sex machines. You may laugh, thinking that I'm crazy, but let's think about it. When you are having sex, your body releases so many happy chemicals! We are the only species on this planet that really enjoys sexual intercourse. We have sex for many different reasons, not just to make babies. We have sex to fall asleep. An orgasm is more powerful than a sleeping pill. We have sex because we are bored. (There don't seem to be any shows we like on the television, and we don't feel like reading a book.) We have sex because we just saw Ocean's 11, and there is enough visual beefcake for a woman to be satisfied for months. Variety is the spice of life. I've heard that some people have sex to keep their significant others from bothering them about last month's credit card bill. This is a morally "grey area," but the reality is their significant other stopped complaining about the bill, didn't they?

Women have sex for many reasons. Perhaps you already knew this, but are you enjoying your sex life? Do you like your body? Could there be improvements? I'm sure every woman answers differently. The truth is you're reading this because you are curious. At some point in every woman's sex life, things can take a downhill turn. (That's if you had an uphill to begin with.) 30% of women have never reached an orgasm. Let me repeat this because this just shouldn't be the case. 30% of women have never had an orgasm! The point of this book is to get you back up the hill or for you 30% out there who need to, to start climbing and reach the top of the orgasm mountain! When your body is in tip-top shape the body takes over and does its thing, just like a well oiled machine. And, when I say tip-top shape I'm not talking "bikini model." I am almost positive that they are not eating right to have an orgasm. You need certain things for your body to be well-oiled, but I will get into that later.

Sex: Whether by yourself or with a partner, this is an important part of looking and feeling amazing. Intercourse improves circulation, breaks up fatty tissue in your body, and improves your immune system function.

Over the years, I have learned that it doesn't matter what you say to try to talk someone out of something when they really want it, or desire it. They will, more than likely, still go after the guy who treats them like dirt, or drink a bottle of wine all by themselves at dinner. Neither of these habits is good for them, and the short and long-term effects can be brutal. No, there is nothing you can do for this friend until they are ready to listen.

So, until you are ready to listen to me, put down this book because nothing I will say will have any meaning to you. But, if you are ready to listen, you will find your world will change. Maybe not your whole universe, but parts of you will grow and develop into the person who you know you can be. We are always changing as people. Sure, there are parts of us that stay the same, but I bet if you give it enough time and attention, those parts will change as well. For example, as a child I hated tomatoes and mayonnaise. I didn't want tomatoes on my salad or in a sandwich. I just couldn't stand it. Now, as an adult I love them, and they are an important part of my diet and well-being. Still, when it comes to mayonnaise, I still don't like it. I can tolerate it if I'm at a summer barbecue (which always seems laden with mayonnaise items!) So, you see, people can change. It's just a matter of when, where, and why.

Back to your mind and your beautiful body! When you are feeling true to yourself, the pounds will start to fall off. It's a combination of you being you, and not caring what people think. When you worry about what people think, you tend not to eat right. I know this because I've been through it. I spent many years trying to change my concern that people's opinions about me matter to me. They just don't, in the long run. Their judgment of you is just that. Judgment, and who are they to judge? I have discovered that people are usually too wrapped up in themselves and how things will affect them, than how they will affect you.

When I was 16, I was sexually assaulted. It was a brutal attack, not just to my body, but to some of the hopes and dreams of what a girl wants to experience when she makes love for the first time. Obviously, this wasn't making love. Love and kindness were nowhere to be seen on that night. Still, what happened happened. I've traveled my path and have grown every step of the way. I would hit bumps along the road, and I would struggle to get over them. One bump in particular was with my body. I was very skinny and tall while growing up. People would stop me on the street and ask if I had an eating disorder. (Why would anyone, and a perfect stranger at that, ask such a personal question?)

I soon discovered that being "me," which was skinny and tall, maybe wasn't the best thing. I even got it into my head that if I wasn't skinny that my assault would have never happened. Anyone who has been through trauma can understand that you go through the "woulda-shoulda-coulda's." I was never someone who cared how many calories were in a piece of chocolate cake. I grew up with parents who taught me to stop eating when I was full. So, I was always healthy no matter how skinny I was. My assault coupled with random people making rude comments to me affected the start of an eating disorder. Instead of starving myself, I started to overeat, and stuff myself with any food in sight. I was determined to be a larger sized girl. The flaw with my new found theory was I have always been active. I was in sports, I loved to dance and walk. I would walk everywhere. I was burning whatever I was eating. This was the beginning of bad food habits. These were new habits, ones that I didn't have as a kid.

I had to retrain my mind that it doesn't matter what people think about how I look. It matters what I think and how I feel. I had to ask myself, why I am I eating this whole bag of chips while watching Grey's Anatomy? Is it boredom? Am I sad? Am I hungry? Am I full? Usually my answer was, because I love barbecue chips! That answer was not good enough, even for this romantic. So, I had to ask again. That lead me to finish fast before I figured out the good answer, and had to put down the bag and pick up an apple! Self control was a constant battle. I still engage in this struggle every day. Sometimes I win, and sometimes I lose! Well, truthfully, I guess I always win in some way, shape, or form.

I am sure you have your own battle to fight. Perhaps it's not with food itself, but all it implies. This is when our wants and our needs collide. These two little guys don't always see eye-to-eye. My desire for a healthy body versus my need for a bag of chips conflicts quite often. In this first phase of the book, I will show you what to eat. This will, in turn, give you the benefits of losing weight (if you really need to,) better skin, shinier hair, longer nails, a sweet tasting little peach (your vagina) and great sex. Some simple foods combined with a little exercise will get you ready for the second phase, The Sexercises. Big Plus: it won't be a major downer, because let's be honest. The second you hear "diet" you automatically run for the hills. It's like a guy hearing the word "marriage!" We all have our individual fear of commitment, it just takes different forms.

What makes me qualified to tell you how to have a better sex life and body by what you eat? Well, I have sex, sometimes with a partner, but I also enjoy this activity with myself. Self love if you will. Mainly, what it comes down to is, I am a woman who really enjoys sexual activity. I am "in love" with being healthy, and want other women to share in this joy. My other qualification is I know what it feels like to not want to eat well, and to stuff your face with all the foods that you think will make you feel better. Eating this way is nice for the moment, but like any one night stand, in the morning you regret it!

Our bodies run on a different kind of love, but so do our individual exercise programs. Much like dating you have to find the right match. For sure, there's going to be the amazing first date and they don't call you ever again. You are left wondering, what did I do? Was it me? Why won't this work?

Then again, there is the person who you've been dating for months and still can't seem to get enough of them. They are perfect! Then, one night you wake up and anything can bother you about them. Like the very fact that they are breathing! As you kneel over him, staring at the drool rolling down his chin, clutching your pillow in both hands, you find yourself wondering whether it's time to silence their snoring, or break up.

It all comes down to the fact that there is a program out there for everyone, and not every program is for you. You should be happy with your choice. It should make you feel and look good. You shouldn't be embarrassed when you introduce your new lifestyle to your friends. They should be looking on in approval asking, "Does it have a brother/sister for me?"

My mother taught us kids a very simple and true rule: when you're full, stop eating. We heard none of the typical, "eat till your plate is clean." That's unhealthy. My siblings and I ate until we were full. We were also fortunate that we grew up in a happy household like this. Food was not about filling an unhappy void. I understand that happens a lot, and I have fallen prey to that in my adulthood. If you learn anything from this book, eat only until you are almost full, and enjoy the healthy food you are consuming.

I know from experience that when you're happy, you eat what is good for you and for your body. When you're unhappy, the opposite occurs. It's almost as if you subconsciously reinforce your unhappiness by making bad food choices. Let's work on getting you to a happier place, and a happier body!

Your Needs

"Serendipity. Look for something, find something else, and realize that what you've found is more suited to your needs than what you thought you were looking for."
- Lawrence Block

There are two things you will need to do:
Change Your Mindset
Find your Motivation

Changing Your Mindset

There comes a point in everyone's life when they say, "Tomorrow, I am going on a diet!" For some people this is a common occurrence. The issue is I am sure you will agree, diets do not work. I take that back. They work for a period of time, but after those few days, weeks or months they fall short of your overall goal. The only successful method is a lifestyle change. Food can be an addiction, plain and simple. You need it to survive. Sometimes it makes you "feel good" and sometimes it cheers you up. Your body is like the child and your mind is like the parent. You have to decide who is in charge, the child or the parent?

The first step is developing an effective mindset. You must love your body the way it is. Right now. Today. This mindset is something you will work on for the rest of your life. No two days in your life are the same. Today you may love your hips. Tomorrow, those hips could be your worst nightmare while wrestling your jeans to the floor after trying to fit them over your thighs. That's part of life. There is no simple way around it. I don't care how thin or heavy, or how tall or short you may be. Every woman, even super models and celebrities, feels bloated and unattractive at times.

I believe we all have something very much in common. We have all had, at one point or another, someone criticize us for how we look, or offer suggestions on how we can improve ourselves. I once had a boyfriend who wanted me to undergo breast augmentation. Obviously, he didn't love me or else he would not have asked me to do such a thing. I don't even have a small "rack" (which wouldn't be a bad thing,) but I'm not a Double D, either. In my opinion, I have an amazing set of lovely lady lumps. When I was living in California, I had people stopping me on the street to ask where I got my breasts "done." Only in Cali right? My reply was always, "God, my friends. God."

When it comes to our body we can become overly critical of ourselves, and of other people. We start to compare our body to someone else's in both positive and negative lights. "Oh, she is stick thin." "Wow, she really gained some weight since I saw her last." "I wish I had her nose."

We are all built differently, and that's what makes us each so beautiful. It's time to see what is beautiful in ourselves and in others. Own and embrace what you have, whatever that may be. Be happy for the person who has a figure like the one you desire. We would live in a better world if we would all love ourselves for whoever that person may be!

I don't believe in trying to change people or trying to mold someone to become the person you want. You love someone through thick and thin. Sure, there may be times when their habits may get on your very last nerve, but you have to choose your battles. (I'm going to go out on a very shaky limb and guess that you're not perfect, either. Who really is?) When it comes to changing ourselves, the only reason to do so is when it's for you, and only you. You are the person who has to live through, and with, any alterations. You have to be strong enough emotionally before any change to your body, mind or spirit can effectively take place. Wanting to grow as a person and human being is always commendable. A tip of the hat to you and your efforts! Just be sure it's for the right reasons.

Amazing Love Diet

Changing your mindset is hard to do in theory, but I think you'll find it easy with just a few pointers. Think about a time in the past when you believed in something strongly, and someone came along who said exactly the right thing to change your mind. Your mind was forever changed, wasn't it? What can you say to yourself that will forever change how you think? One way I have found to change my mindset is to decide that my body and I are in a romantic relationship. This isn't hard for my mind to believe in since, typically in the past, I was single and the only action I got was with myself! It's not that farfetched for me to convince my body that we are in a relationship. There are moments when it would seem we're in an abusive relationship, but I am always working on the balance! When you are in a loving, healthy relationship, don't you want that person to live forever? Aren't you planning on spending the rest of your life with them?

For example, one ex ate like he couldn't care any less whether he lived or died. When I started to believe we had some form of a future together, I started to freak out. I didn't want this guy to die on me, leaving me with five kids, a mortgage, and no sex! I immediately started incorporating salads and fresh fruit into his diet.

Ex-boyfriend's first reaction, "What's this green stuff? Ugh and why does it taste like grass?"

The answer was simple, "It's tastes like grass because it is grass. Kind of. I want to make sure we grow old together, which I'm afraid isn't going to happen if you continue eating the way you do."

Ex-boyfriend's reply, "If you keep feeding me stuff like this, there isn't going to be a future for us either."

That's where I learned that there is a delicate balance between eating healthy and treating yourself. The two must live in harmony, never feeling like the one is taking over the other. When it came down to it, my ex and I were opposites. I was healthy and he was like a treat. This relationship didn't last because the treat didn't want the balance of being healthy. If you can learn to keep your romantic relationships healthy and in balance, you are on the right path for your body, too.

If you find your romantic relationships lacking in the healthy and balanced department, then may I suggest changing your mindset to believe that your body is a child. Would you feed a child a whole container of pre-made cookie dough? No, you would have a fun day making cookies and then after you ate your dinner, you would have some as a treat. When your "child" has been good, such as putting up with co-workers all week, or you've been to the gym three times this week, you may reward yourself with a fancy dinner and a glass of wine.

Change your mind set. Instead of thinking of how many calories are in the piece of chocolate cake, think about what would you give your child? Are you going to give your child that piece of cake? Possibly. Is it a special occasion like a birthday or wedding? Have you been eating so well that you just want to treat yourself? Are you too tired from work and you can't find the energy to make a proper dinner, and there is already a cake made up, just waiting on the table for a nibble? In my opinion, all reasons are valid. Sometimes it's a special occasion. Sometimes life is a celebration in itself, and sometimes it takes all your energy just to pick up the fork. I would like to believe you would feed your child in moderation. An example of a great rule my sister and her husband have come up with for their family is: Treats on Wednesdays and Saturdays. But, when any of the grandparents are around and want to give the kids treats, then it's ok. This rule is wonderful. It keeps you feeling like you get something for all your hard work, everything is still in good balance, and every now and then you'll feel spoiled.

Having a treat and being "spoiled" every now and then brings us to "cheating." What is it? Figure out how cheating is defined in your mind when it comes to your diet and don't do it, plain and simple. We all make sacrifices. When one gets married or is in a committed relationship, you make a promise to be true to your partner. You're committed to your body aren't you? The ground rules are set for what is considered cheating. Of course you're still going to enjoy life. Commitment is not a death sentence. You love the Opera and your partner doesn't? Not a bad thing, just go with a friend. You love fried chicken. Find a recipe that is still healthy but can satisfy your craving. If there are no healthy recipes out there for you, then now it's considered a treat. That means, have the fried chicken in moderation.

Find something that can satisfy your cravings without derailing you from your overall health goals. What can you live with, and what can't you live without? "Let your conscience be your guide," as my father would always say.

Motivation

What motivates you? What do you think will keep you motivated? To keep up with any health or exercise regimen, you need to have some form of motivation. It can be difficult to get to the gym. We are all busy and maybe even a little nervous. Sometimes it can be hard to keep the momentum going when we take breaks from our diet and fitness activities. Maybe we didn't do anything physical this past week or we skipped our spin/yoga/ stripper pole class. I've observed that many persons stop working out after a few days of "taking a break." Life becomes too busy and hectic and we say to ourselves, "I'll do it tomorrow." Next thing you know, a week has gone by, and we don't even know where our sneakers are hiding. Breaks are fine; just get yourself doing something after the time out. Even just one activity can get your mind back into taking care of your body.

Here are some motivators that I have been hearing from people lately.

I WANT TO:
Eat whatever I want
Wear whatever I want
Wear a strapless dress

I have a wedding or reunion coming up
It's bikini season
Vacation next month!

I want to set a good example for my children
I have health concerns
My body/heart/soul/psyche needs to heal

For me, one of my major motivators is love. I stay in shape for my significant other, and for the love of myself. It's a great motivator for my love not to want to take their eyes and hands off of me! If that means doing an extra Pilates session or even just 10 more minutes on the treadmill, I'm there. I also try to eat as healthily as possible for the love of my body, mind and soul. For me, sticking as close as I can to a clean diet, with no processed foods, is essential.

Now, when I'm not in a relationship, motivations become more short term and mainly support a pleasurable and satisfying life. Staying in shape so that I can eat as much as I want between Thanksgiving and New Years is a big one! Getting my butt to the gym because I'm going on vacation is another. Again, the focus is eating whatever I want. I'm a pleasure seeker. Good food, good wine and good love are my main focuses and motivations in life.

We all have moments when we feel unbelievably beautiful. Unfortunately, we also have moments when we feel disgusted with ourselves, and we vow to never again to finish a tub of ice cream in one sitting! Next time, we will take our time and finish it in two. It's a balancing act to stay healthy and happy. Sometimes the two do not mesh together easily, but certainly they should work together for the good of the body. For your ultimate success, your goals are to have a different mindset, and to have some form of motivation.   In this phase, these are your only needs. Everything else will fall into place once you change your mindset and are motivated.

Dieting Around the World

"In spite of food fads, fitness programs, and health concerns, we must never lose sight of a beautifully conceived meal."
- Julia Child

Traveling, meeting new people and experiencing a new culture are passions of mine. I love waking up in a new city or town and not knowing all of the possibilities that await me outside my bedroom doors. I have yet to travel this whole world, so there is much for me yet to learn and to see. I have met many women (a few men) along my journey who I call my Mothers. They have taken me in when I needed a mother, since I was more than likely far away from my own little Mother. I have put together some of the diet tips they taught me in my travels.   The one diet secret that was in common with all of my mothers from around the world: Life is to be enjoyed, and is too short for a diet!

Please remember this one diet secret, even if you don't remember anything else: Remember that life is to be enjoyed and is too short to not love life for all its splendors. Live like you only have this moment, but also take care of your body like you're going to live till 100.

French Mother: Drink Wine and Eat Good Fats.
It was early morning when I arrived in Brussels via a London train. This was my first time in Brussels. I was to stay with my cousin's friend, who became my French Mother. My eyes were sleepy but my heart was pounding with excitement. The city of Brussels was hustling and bustling. The sun was just coming up over this historic place. I arrived at my French Mother's townhouse and started to unpack. "This is all you have?" she asked me.

I try to travel light whenever I can. I also wanted to be able to bring a little something back to the States for my family and friends. Can't do a tour of Europe and not have at least a little gift for the ones you love! Every moment I got to spend with my French Mother was a delight. She was so smart and knowledgeable. I felt a connection with her instantly. Every night I would get home from my exploring and she would be cooking something so scrumptious I could hardly contain myself. Most of the meal's ingredients had been purchased just that day which is what you do in Europe. You always purchase fresh food every day. Every night during my visit with her we would talk about everything until very late in the evening. We would both realize what time it was and decide to get some sleep. In truth, I wanted to talk to her all night long. And when it came time for me to leave, I really didn't want to. I think of her always. Even though we only spent a few days together, she has had an enormous impact on my life. I will never be the same Dorothy again. For one of our meals she opened my eyes to Raclette, which is something the Swiss enjoy during their winter season. The set up is as follows: There is a special grill with multiple small pans that will be used to melt the slices of cheese. Once the cheese is melted and wonderfully gooey, pour over potatoes. My French Mother taught me an important lesson that day. "Never, ever, drink water when you are eating melted cheese. When the cheese and the water combined in your stomach you will end up with a terrible stomach ache because it is hard for the water to break down the cheese. Drink wine. The acidity in the wine helps to break down the cheese, which makes digestion easier." She didn't have to tell me twice to drink wine. I was all over it. "I drink a glass or two as often as I can. My husband knows more about wine than I do. I just love to drink it."

My French Mother also taught me to have a bit of good fat before each meal. A spoonful of olive oil or some nuts will do the trick.

Benefits of drinking wine

Reduces risk of death At least, most causes of mortality. Red wine has a protective effect on your body. Heart Disease It is well known that having a glass of red wine a day can keep the heart doctor away. Red wine reduces production of LDL (low density lipoprotein) and boosts HDL (high density lipoprotein) cholesterol.

Atherosclerosis: Not here! This is hardening of the arteries, usually caused when blood vessels are no longer able to relax. Red wine can help to relax blood vessels and help promote healthy blood flow.

Alzheimer's disease and Aging: There is a lower risk of Alzheimer's disease. Resveratrol is found in red wine, which can protect your brain and body against aging.

Heart Attacks: Having up to two glasses a day for women, and up to three a day if you're a man, can reduce your risk for a heart attack. Red wine can help a person to de-stress, which puts less strain on the heart.

Now, if you are someone who doesn't drink, you are still able to receive red wine's benefits. Here are a few ways: Eating red grapes on a regular basis. The skin of grapes contains many nutrients and antioxidants, just like the juice of the fruit.   Peanuts also contain Resveratrol. These little nuts have a slightly higher amount of Resveratrol than grapes!

Remember, everything in moderation. This does not mean if you miss your glass of wine on Sunday, you can have three on Monday! Sorry, but it just doesn't work that way. If you are someone who is watching your weight, I suggest that instead of dessert you may have a glass of red wine.

If you don't already drink, there isn't a need to start. You may find yourself with a bad habit or gaining unwanted pounds since alcohol is "empty calories."

Benefits of good fats

Not only are good fats great for your hair, skin and nails, but good fats helps to stabilize cholesterol, improve the body's immune system and helps you to stay fuller longer. This aids in weight-loss, or at the very least, in stabilizing weight and overall health of the body. Even though good fats are good, remember that fats are still fats. So, everything in moderation. Just a few almonds before each meal will help you to lose weight and make you feel great!

Vietnamese Mother: Drink Tea and Eat Dark Chocolate

I woke up to the din of a crowd of voices. I thought, 'there must be a party going on downstairs!" I was staying with my one of my best friends, KitKat. I walked down the stairs to see what all the commotion was. I entered a small living room and about five of KitKat's little cousins where playing. Their mouths dropped open when they saw me. Standing at 5'10", I was by far the tallest person in the house at that moment. From the look on KitKat's cousins' faces, I may have been the first person of my height in this house, ever!

"Hello!" I gave a little wave. "Where is KitKat?" Their mouths still hadn't sprung back into place and they continued to stare at me. "Ok...well nice to see you. I'll go find her."

I walked into the kitchen where KitKat was watching her family play a card game. Everyone turned to me and gave me an up-and-down once over. I felt more awkward than usual and having just awakened, I wondered if my face had the imprint of the pillow and if my eyes had eye goo in them. Then, my Vietnamese Mother, KitKat's mother, ran right up to me and gave me a big hug. "How was your nap? Are you hungry? I'll make you something. Here, have some tea first. Prepares the body to eat."

As I sipped on my tea, I was introduced to the whole family. Well, the small portion of the family who was at the house that day. I heard an aunt say something in Vietnamese. KitKat turned to me and said, "She said you look like Jessica Simpson." I quickly smiled, since I think Jessica is beautiful, "Thank you!"

Whenever I visit KitKat her family is so welcoming and warm. Her mother and father always offer me something to eat when I enter their home. It makes me feel like I'm back with my family. Sometimes, KitKat will protest in Vietnamese, while her Mother is trying to feed me one of her special dishes, "No, Mother, we are leaving soon. We're going to eat out tonight." I just smile and nod but part of me wants to stay in and eat her mother's cooking. It's beyond tasty and healthy. Plus, how can I say no to the special shrimp dish she makes?

While watching a movie with KitKat, my Vietnamese Mother will come in to check on us and see if there is anything that we need. "Would you like some soup? I will pour you some tea." She will leave the room and come back with tea for the both of us and a bowl of chocolates to share. "It's dark chocolate. I eat this every day, keeps me young and healthy and it makes me smile." Her Mother says, overjoyed.

KitKat's mother is maybe the sweetest woman on the planet, and probably the cutest. Aside from her disposition, she is a very smart little mother and keeps her family eating well. Through her cooking she has a very healthy, satisfied, and happy family indeed.

Benefits of drinking tea

Drinking tea before you begin to consume food will help prepare the body for digestion. Tea also may aid in the body's elimination of waste and toxins. Tea also contains anti-oxidants, boosts immune system in the blood, and boosts metabolism. Drinking five cups a day of green tea can help one to burn up to 80 additional calories.

Benefits of eating dark chocolate daily

There are benefits to eating dark chocolate. I suggest around three ounces a day. Not only do you get your chocolate fix, and I'm sure that will put a smile on your face, but chocolate may help you to lose weight. Eating something sweet like fruit or chocolate sends a signal to the brain that you are full and the meal is complete. Dark chocolate increases endorphin production. When a female eats chocolate it stimulates the same pleasure section in the brain as sex does. Chocolate may also be an anti-depressant since it contains serotonin. Also, dark chocolate has a small amount of caffeine, which helps to ease PMS issues.

Italian Mother: Olive Oil

"I have olive oil with every meal. Everyone in my family loves olive oil. It's a staple. We dip bread in it, we cook with it and we even drink it. Olive oil is life." My Italian Mother is everything you would want in an "Italian Mother." She is warm, a great cook and has great fashion sense. I've noticed that Europeans have a way of speaking and conversing that makes life that much more beautiful. They really do know how to enjoy life, at least it would seem this way. Their priorities are different than those of Americans. Americans want wealth and fame and we want it yesterday. Everything is so fast for us. I found in Italy, life is fast, but in a different way. It's a land where eating habits become social, family is number one, and driving slowly is not optional!

One of my favorite moments with my Italian Mother was when we went shopping. Actually, we weren't supposed to be shopping. We were supposed to be meeting up with the family and we were late. "Ok, Hun, we have less than ten minutes. Stick with me, I'll show you how it's done." We continued into the store and my Italian Mother moved with fury. Never have I seen anyone move that fast and still be that graceful. She was like a lioness hunting her prey. She picked out a few items she liked and moved right to the check-out. We were in and out in less than ten minutes. I was impressed and vowed I would learn all that I could from this woman.

She taught me hints about many things: How to make a yummy, gooey lasagna, how to choose the right man ("He has to love you more than anything my dear!") and about olive oil. "Olive oil is life," as my Italian Mother has said. She typically will have a spoonful in the morning, a spoonful when she's hungry but can't eat yet, and a spoonful before bed.

Benefits of Olive Oil
Olive oil is great for the skin, hair and nails. It has been known for centuries that this oil can slow the aging process and help with arthritis. This oil also contains other health benefits. If you have a spoonful of olive oil when you wake up, and have another spoonful before bed, it will help aid the body's elimination process of waste and toxins. If you are ever feeling hungry, this oil will actually help you to curb your hunger and cravings. So, when you are reaching for pint of ice cream, maybe fill your spoon up first with some olive oil. Wait a minute for your brain to realize its full, and hopefully you won't overdo it on the Chunky Monkey. All of these benefits are key to a healthy, fit body.

Mexican Mother: Love and Avocados
"I tell those I love that I love them. Americans hold back the telling of love, when they shouldn't." One of my boyfriends, who grew up in Mexico, and I were together for only one week before he told me he loved me, and I told him I loved him. It was normal. In America, if you tell someone that you love them they run away, even though they may love you back. Makes no sense. No wonder

Americans have more cases of illness. You hold everything in. You don't share the happy moments and you stew in the sad moments. "Things happen, Dorotee. Life happens. All we have is love." This is what my Mexican Mother said to me on one of our first encounters. I knew then, we were always going to be in each other's lives. She is younger than I am, but age doesn't matter when it comes to the heart. She is always there for me, protecting me, and if needs be, fighting for me. That sounds like a mother to me. Her key to staying healthy is eating good-for-you food like avocados, putting love into all of her cooking, and saying "I love you" to who she loves every day, as many times a day as she can.

Benefits of Avocados

Avocados contain the good fats that we love for healthy hair, skin and nails. Healthy fats also help one to lose weight. Avocados also contain vitamin E which is essential to the body's health. Avocados have been known to help prevent cancer, especially prostate, breast and oral cancers. So, maybe it's time to have an avocado a day. I don't know about you, but I love fresh guacamole.

Benefits of saying "I love you"

Saying I love you to someone actually helps to form a bond between the two persons. Endorphins are released in both persons' brains when you say or hear "I love you." Saying I love you is both beneficial to the person saying this phrase, but also beneficial to the person receiving it. This simple phrase may boost your immune system as well as boost your metabolism. These benefits aid in weight-loss as well as over-all body function and health. So, start telling those you love that you love them...everyday...all day!

Portuguese Mother: Eat Little Meals, Be Social and Take Your Time

"When I eat it's because I need to eat. I need the food that I am about to put in my body. When I go out to eat, it's an experience. I'm there to be with friends and family. If I'm by myself, I'm there to be with myself and enjoy my own company. I take my time. There is no rush to get back to work because the work will still be there when I get back to my office. You Americans, everything is so fast, so quick. You are all in such a rush to eat. You don't actually experience what you are eating. What is the point of eating, if you're just going to gobble up your meal? No, I take my time and enjoy my meal. Enjoy time with my family and friends. What is the point to life anyway? Are we put on this earth to slave away all day at a desk? I hope not."

I met my Portuguese Mother while visiting Oporto, Portugal. It is a city that still closes down on Sundays and most businesses are small, family-owned-and-run. She helped me out quite a bit while I was visiting her city: She told me what sites to see, where to eat, and how to make a group of dogs stop following me around the city. This last tip was extra helpful since I was a few moments away from adopting each puppy and   bringing them back to the states with me!

There was one restaurant in particular that she shared with me. It was around the corner from where I was staying. As I was deciding on what I was going to have for dinner, she told me how her family eats. "Only eat a little bit at a time. You take one bite and put down your fork or spoon. Chew your food, listen to the conversation, have a sip of wine. Then you may take another bite and start the process all over again. Don't rush your meal and pay attention to what is going on around you. If you don't you could miss something." She also told me that taking a nap everyday was the key to good health. "It's not just for babies. Everyone needs a nap."

Benefits of eating slowly

When one eats slowly it allows more time for the brain to send the "full" signal to the stomach to stop eating.

This allows your body to only consume what it needs in the way of substance. So, eat slowly. You will eat fewer calories which will aid in weight-loss, or will result in no weight gain. Also, one will take the time to enjoy the food that is placed before them. Enjoy your food, enjoy your life.

Benefits of Taking a Nap

There are so many health benefits to taking a cat nap that I am really surprised that it's not part of our everyday life. In fact, I sense that it's frowned upon in the states to take a nap. The belief seems to be that you are lazy for taking a nap. The benefits, in my opinion, outweigh the dirty looks you will receive. Taking a cat nap reduces stress, and aids in heart health. A nap allows you the time to stay focused at work and boosts creativity. Napping also burns calories and allows the body to have a higher rate of cell turnover. So, if you want a slimmer waistline, less stress in your life, and better skin? Take a cat nap.

Brazilian Mother: Pineapple

I met my Brazilian Mother while shopping one day. Actually, my Brazilian Mother isn't a woman, but a gay man. He isn't offended when I call him my Brazilian Mother. On the contrary, he likes it when I call him Hot Momma. He helped me pick out a pair of shoes and a dress for a party that I was attending. During the minutes between finding out my shoe size (size 7) and finding out my dress size (size 6) we became friends. Not sure how I reeled this little 5'5" Brazilian hottie in, but I am so happy that I did. Not only has he helped me fashion-wise, but he has opened my eyes to many diet secrets that have helped me to stay slim. At the top of the list? Eating pineapple after a meal. "Giselle does this, baby. Everyone in Brazil does this, baby." I have no idea if Giselle eats pineapple. She could be allergic to pineapple for all I know. His Brazilian accent is very thick, which for some reason makes me believe that Giselle does eat pineapple after every meal! How else could she stay so thin after eating a hamburger and fries for lunch?

Benefits of Eating Pineapple

Pineapples contain Bromelain which is an enzyme that aids digestion. One may take a Bromelain tablet instead of fresh pineapple, and this should be taken in between meals to aid digression. Pineapple also contains vitamin C which boosts immune system function and helps with anti-aging. My suggestion is to eat pineapple in between meals as a healthy snack. Do not eat with other foods in order to receive the full benefits.

Irish Mother: Bananas and Laugh All Day

I had met my Irish Mother while I was playing with a child I was babysitting. We hit it off right away. She has such a great laugh and smile, they're infectious. One day while we were catching up at her house, she told me about her large family back in Ireland. "All we do is laugh! Oh we love beer, but who doesn't love beer?" She said this to me in a slight Irish brogue. Being in the states for as long as she has been, she's lost most of her accent. The only time I would hear it come out in full force was when I went with her to Ireland and spent some time with her beautiful family. While catching up with my Irish Mother, she said she was going to make herself a smoothie, did I want one as well? I never pass on a smoothie, so I said yes please! She started to prepare the smoothie and turned to me, "You know I started putting a banana in my smoothies. I've noticed that when I do, I feel fuller longer. It could just be in my head, but I have noticed a change in my hunger and how I act throughout the day. I don't eat as much. Do you want a banana in your smoothie?" I thought about it for a moment and decided to try my own experiment. "Yes please. Thank you for the smoothie!"

We enjoyed our smoothie and laughed the afternoon away until it was time for me to head home for dinner. My first thought when I arrived at my house was, "Oh my goodness, I'm not hungry and I have plenty of energy. I may even go for a run." Then I remembered I don't like to run, so I went for a walk on the beach instead.

Benefits of Laughing

Laughing speeds your heart rate, releases muscle tension, and increases the amount of oxygen in your blood. It also produces the happy drug in the brain called endorphins. In theory, if you laughed for 15 minutes every day, you'd burn enough calories to lose one pound a year. Laughing burns 1.5 calories per minute. So the more you laugh, the more weight you will lose. That is amazing!

Benefits of Bananas

Not only does a banana help in making a smoothie thicker and creamer, but it also contains health benefits. The biggest benefit that most people already know is that bananas contain potassium. Potassium aids in the body's overall health, especially with heart function. Bananas also help to stabilize your mood. Bananas contain the highest amount of B6, which helps to stablize blood sugars. Bananas contain fiber. Add bananas to your breakfast, combined with a nutbutter for a midday snack, or add it to your fruit smoothie.

My French Great-Grandmother: Eat Fresh, Clean Foods

I wasn't named after Dorothy from Oz. I was named after my great-grandmother, Dorothy, or "Ma" as the rest of my family and I refers to her. She is a little French woman standing at 4'9" with hair and heels. Just the cutest thing you have ever seen. I remember walking into her house when I was younger and seeing her vacuum in stiletto heels. I thought to myself, "I want to be like that!" For years now, when anyone would speak to my Ma she would just smile, nod and say "Yes". She has had trouble hearing for quite some time now. She's didn't want to be disagreeable. It wouldn't matter what you were saying to her, she would just smile and nod so very sweetly.

My Ma's backyard was full of flowers and shade trees, but the majority of the backyard was a large fruit and vegetable garden. The freshest, tastiest fruits and vegetables came from my Ma's garden. Ma was quite the gardener. To this day, her homemade pickles can't be beat and her tomatoes are the juiciest. Nothing compares to her homemade strawberry jam. In her younger years, if she didn't grow it, then she didn't eat it. She grew up during the Great Depression, when food and money were scarce. She learned at a young age to grow and can her own fruits and vegetables. Some say because she didn't grow up with processed foods, this was the reason for her living so long. She was healthy and was able to stay independent until just a few months before she passed away at the age of 99.

Benefits of eating fresh fruits and vegetables

Fresh fruits and veggies are a must for weight-loss and overall body health. Not only do fresh fruits and veggies contain fiber, but some actually contain protein, such as peas. Start your own little garden today. Nothing tastes as good as your own fresh tomato sauce. Plus, the money saved from having your own garden will allow you to take a trip, or to treat yourself to a manicure!

Gardening is also a great stress reliever for some people. It allows you time in the sun (Vitamin D) and a way to be with nature. It also is a great way to feel like you have accomplished something. While I lived in San Diego, I had a mini garden on my balcony. I grew herbs and some veggies. I was so proud of myself when my first cucumber showed up. Honestly, it felt like I could accomplish anything after that. Funny, how growing your own food will do that to your ego.

Benefits of Clean Foods (Not processed)

The benefits of having a clean diet not only extend to weight-loss, but also to your hair, skin and nails. The chemicals in processed foods may dull skin and hair. Once you cut out anything processed, your body's weight will stabilize, you will have more energy, and you may even find you have a happier disposition and attitude.

Benefits of Making Your Own Junk Food

I do not know many people who are able to stay completely away from junk food. So, what about making your own? They will not have as many chemicals and won't be as processed as store-bought. Start making your own potato chips, cookies and ice cream. You may find a new outlet for stress (I find when I bake, I am at peace with myself.) You will be helping to keep you and your loved ones healthy, as well as satisfied.

My Own Mother: Dessert

Growing up we didn't eat a lot of junk. Every now and again my parents would order a pizza and we were allowed to have a glass of soda. We didn't eat or drink this type of food on a regular basis. I don't even remember going to any fast food places as a child, only when we asked for our birthday parties to be at any particular fast food chain. It wasn't normal to eat junk. When I wanted a snack my Mother would say, "Have a piece of fruit or a piece of cheese." My Mother cooked well-balanced meals for all of us (six) children and my 6'6" tall father. She did, however, have dessert treats for us! These treats were always homemade. It was way too expensive for her to do it any other way when I was a child. For six little scavengers you had to watch the food budget. A phrase I recall hearing from my father was, "If it's healthy, then kids probably don't want to eat it. So, find out what the kids hate and give them plenty of it." My Mother's only rule when it came to us eating treats was, "If you have a little bit of dinner, then you may have a little bit of dessert." I often remember asking what we were having for dinner, and if I wasn't happy with the answer, quickly following up with, "What are we having for dessert?" Sometimes this rang true with what my Mother cooked. Healthy, well balanced meals. So, if I knew we were going to have a tasty dessert then I could handle dinner.

Five Year Old Self: "I'm full."
Parents: "Just a few more bites."
Five Year Old Self: "Ok, may I have dessert?"
Father: "You said you were full."
Five Year Old Self: "Well, I'm full from dinner, but I left this much room for dessert." (I put my hands into a small circle and placed it on my belly.)

Benefits of Balancing Dinner and Dessert

I don't know about you, but there are times when I am not in the mood for a regular dinner, I want a piece of chocolate cake. Knowing that I am in the mood for dessert, I try to keep that in mind when I am planning my dinner. I plan on eating enough to get the nutrients that I need for a healthy body and then leave room for dessert. This is a delicate balance since how do you know how much room will be needed for that yummy piece of chocolate cake? Eat slowly and have time between dinner and dessert. This allows your brain plenty of time to determine how much dessert that the body will be able to handle without stuffing your body and making you have that icky feeling of over-eating. My Mother's rule of thumb, if you have a little bit of dinner than you may have a little bit of dessert. So if you only have half a salad and a piece of chicken. For dessert you may have 3oz of dark chocolate. Per what my Father would always say to my siblings and me, "Let your conscience be your guide." It's a nice rule of thumb for sure.

Scandinavia Mother: Eat Whatever, and Enjoy Talking About Sex, and Having Sex

"Sex is so taboo in America. You Americans are how do you say...Prudes? It's not a big deal to talk about sex, to walk around naked, or to have sex. It's natural. From a young age, we are taught our bodies are natural and beautiful. If a man sees your breasts at the beach, it's not a big deal. He doesn't stare and make you feel uncomfortable." My response was, "Well, maybe it's good that we Americans are more prudish. Whenever my old boyfriend would see my breasts, his eyes would bulge right out of his head and he would say it felt like Christmas. Can't beat that compliment!"

My Scandinavia Mother has a rock solid body, is over 40, and a blonde, blue eyed beauty. She doesn't "work out" and she doesn't "diet." What does she do to stay to healthy? "I live life and I eat well. I don't deny myself something I want. If I want pasta, I eat pasta. I don't work out, but I go swimming or find some other activity I enjoy." Maybe it's her good genes, but I have a sneaky suspicion that it's her outlook and her energy that keeps her looking so amazing.

Benefits of Sex

Sex is by far my favorite subject. I love to talk about it. For me, it is completely normal to discuss sex, since it is one of my passions and obsessions. Sex is healthy. Sex is natural. The benefits of sex are so long I could write a whole book on just sex alone. (Maybe I will.) Not only does sex provide great exercise for toning your muscles and burning calories, but on average, sex burns about 300 calories in an hour. This includes kissing, foreplay and intercourse, oh my. Intercourse is a great way to stretch and tone your whole body, sometimes muscles you didn't even realize that you had. If you're feeling guilty about eating that piece of cake or that pound of bacon, maybe it's time to grab your honey and do the "No Pants Dance". Or just dance by yourself. That burns calories and tones your body as well. You don't need a partner to get the benefits of sex.

Benefits of Eating What You Want

For me, when I've been on diets in the past and I'm not allowed to eat a certain food or have a particular drink, that food or beverage becomes all I can think about. When one limits oneself, you destroy free will and your freedom to do what brings you joy in this world. While it is true everything should be in moderation, knowing that it makes you gain weight also may help not feeling sad about not being able to eat a certain food. Think of it as being allergic to the food that causes you to gain weight. Listen to your body. I know that I love beer, but it makes me feel sick, and causes my stomach to blow up like a balloon. I try to stay away from beer as much as possible, even though sometimes that's all I want to drink on a hot summer day. Eat what you want, but know that there are limits when it comes to your body and your overall health.

Eat, Drink & Be Merry

"Nothing would be more tiresome than eating and drinking if God had not made them a pleasure as well as a necessity."

-Voltaire

There was a moment in my life when I realized that, sometimes, food is better than sex, or at the very least, it's comparable. I was having dinner with my one of my best friends. My closest friends and I share many of the same interests. We enjoy the great pleasures in life. The consumption of good food and great wine is something we enjoy together. I don't really remember what myself and this particular friend had to eat that night, but it was incredible. I'm sure we started with one or two amazing appetizers followed up with a tantalizing fish entrée, and an amazing bottle of red wine. My friend is very good at choosing wine. She learned by traveling and tasting wines all over the world.

We finished our meals with a smoldering, chocolate lava cake oozing with chocolaty goodness. After the last bite, we both sat back quite sated, and looked at each other, not saying a word. It was one of the best meals either of us had ever had and words could not describe the joy our bodies were feeling. It wasn't just a meal but was a completely satisfying experience in so many ways, at least for me. I can't speak for my friend, but judging from the look on her face, she felt the same way as I did. For another several minutes, I don't think we moved. We couldn't. Our bodies had released so many happy endorphins and euphoric feelings that our minds had to shut down in order to take it all in. Honestly, I don't know if I could handle having a meal like that every day. My body would go into stimulated overload because of the pure joy my taste buds would be feeling.

It was comparable to some of my best orgasms. You know the kind, or if you don't you soon will, where after you can't move, think or speak. Sometimes you have enough energy to listen or feel your own heartbeat beating quickly in your chest, and you take in a deep breath to try to collect yourself. But, that's all that your mind can handle at that moment in time. This feeling was that meal.

Couldn't move, couldn't speak, and certainly I was completely satisfied. It was most definitely a multiple-orgasmic meal, if you will.

This got me to thinking. If food could cause multiple orgasms of the taste buds in our mouths, then perhaps this could be a major reason why some women who are so unsatisfied sexually turn to food. Heck, I would, and sometimes do! There are two men in this world who have never let me down, and who can always satisfy a craving or two: Ben and Jerry. Curling up with them and a romantic movie is a great night to me. That is, of course, until I start not fitting into my jeans. That's when that relationship goes sour. We start to fight. I say, never again will I be fooled by you, never again. Really? Food can be a love/hate relationship, but it doesn't have to be. You can have your cake and eat it too! Just not all at once, and not all the time

When I think "diet," I think of a quick fix. When I hear "lifestyle change," I hear big commitment and torture. From my observation, most people have similar beliefs. Isn't there a healthy routine that doesn't require me giving up everything I love, all for the sake of a conventional "perfect" body? I was overjoyed for my body, my soul and my mind when I found it. I could love my body inside and out, and reach the goals I was so desperately trying to obtain with greater success than I had had in the past.

Treating your body with love is the key to a healthy body. Example: If you are pregnant, and are committed with love to have a healthy baby, you will do all the things you're supposed to do when you're pregnant to ensure that end. You eat non-processed foods, lots of fruit and veggies, lean proteins, and take your daily vitamins. If you take that approach with your body, thinking of this as a "gestational" project, you'll find your body is "developing" into shape and you look and feel great.

What would you feed your child? Most parents want their children to eat what is best for them, but the parent herself may tend to skip meals, eat unhealthy foods, and or to eat on the run. Do you want your children to develop unhealthy eating habits? I would hope not. The best way to ensure that your child eats healthily is to monitor what they consume. My suggestion is to do the same for you. When growing up, it was only on special occasions like birthdays or holidays that we were allowed to consume unhealthy portions of foods. We always had dessert. If we just ate a little dinner, then we got a little dessert. It was balanced. (The exceptions were anytime a grandparent gave us ice cream for breakfast, and the night we decorated our Christmas tree!)

When it comes to breaking a habit, all we are really doing is starting up another (hopefully healthy) habit to take its place. An example: substitute dark chocolate for milk chocolate. It's higher in antioxidants.

There is no right time to start a diet, but there are always plenty of excuses not to: "If I start now, I'll miss all the holiday parties." Or, my favorite, "After this weekend, I'll start my diet." You will always fail with this attitude. Just start now. Doesn't mean you give up on carbs and wine altogether. Just consume these treats in moderation. Are you heading to a big party this Saturday? Perfect! Have a game plan before you put on your party dress. That's why I take my eating experiences as they come, one day at a time. Just because you're not on a conventional diet doesn't mean you shouldn't eat well today, or that it gives you a free pass to eat whatever you want, anytime you want. You are alive aren't you? Time to act like it! What you put in your mouth should be for a very good reason. There is a way to balance eating healthy and eating happy.

I have mentioned before about motivation and love. When it comes to most of what I eat I eat certain foods knowing they are going to help my love life. Everything is connected. And I mean this in every sense of the word. If you eat a piece of fruit, it nourishes your body. It makes its way through your system and provides your body with the benefits of vitamins, pectin for your arteries' health, and wonderful fiber. But, this piece of fruit helps in other ways as well. I am sure you've heard of aphrodisiacs, right? Certain foods help to turn you on and get you in the mood for sex. Well, this is true! But, did you also know there are foods that can make sex better for you and your partner, as well as make you look more attractive?

Here is a list of foods that help your body as a sexual being:

Fats

Olive oil, Grapeseed Oil, Avocado oil, Avocados, Chia seeds and flax seed. These are great, and rich in the types of healthy fats you want for your skin and hair. They help to get the blood flowing to the right areas, if you know what I mean.

Fruits
Any fruit is good for your body, but these are the best:
Fruit sweetens you literally. You will have a sweeter taste and smell in your nether region.
Apples - Great benefits
Strawberries
Oranges - Great benefits
Grapes
Apricots
Bananas
Peaches

Veggies and Legumes
These are the best! Bright colors, as well as green, are best for your sexual body.

Avocado
Carrots - Helps to give you a great glow and it is a natural at fighting harmful rays from the sun.
Celery - Great for your bones. It is said that the resulting smell your skin will secrete makes you more attractive sexually.
Cucumbers
Eggplant
Tomato
Beans
Garlic
Leeks
Onions
Peppers
Soybeans
Spinach
Sweet potatoes
Lentils
Beets
Winter squash

Protein
Some vegetables and grains contain protein. The best sources of protein, in my opinion, are fish, beans, eggs, lean chicken or turkey. If you love meat like steak and burgers, keep these to twice a month, maybe when you are feeling yourself getting weak, or if you just love meat and need to meet a craving. Too much red meat causes the taste of your genitals and skin to be bitter and sour.

Salmon is the best
Sardines, if you can stand them
Seafood, Shrimp, Scallops, Oysters (Oysters have a special power. It is not true what they say about them being an aphrodisiac, but they will help you to climax faster)
Eggs, egg yolks are great for you.
Eel (If you like sushi)
Kidney beans

Black beans
Soy
Tofu
Seeds: Pine nuts and pumpkin
Nuts like cashews, almonds and walnuts

Grains
Your grains are not limited to just the following. I love quinoa and I think it is such a power food.
Quinoa
Brown Rice
Steal Cut Oats

What to drink
Lots of water to flush out your system, and to keep your skin hydrated and glowing
Teas such as green, white or nettle (Nettle tea has certain qualities that aid the vagina's scent)
Alcohol dulls the skin, but having a glass of red wine has many benefits and those benefits increase during the hours of happy hour, believe it or not. Having a glass between the hours of 4-8 is a good thing. (But, why limit "Happy" to just an hour?)

Miscellaneous

Benefits of Chia Seeds:

-Makes you feel fuller longer: So if you don't want to add calories but you want to feel full and have health benefits this is your magic food.
-Balance Blood Sugar: Slows down the body's conversion of starches into sugars.
-Omega-3s and 6: By weight, Chia seeds contains more omega 3 than salmon and flax seeds.
-Protein: 1 tablespoon of Chia seeds contains 2 grams of protein. Chia seeds are a complete protein, so no need to combine with other foods.
-Fiber: 1 tablespoon contains 5.5 grams of fiber

-Fight Aging: Chia seeds are packed with anti-oxidants.
-Vitamins: Contains calcium, magnesium, copper, iron, zinc and many more!
-Easy to Digest: Unlike flax seeds these beauties don't need to be ground up. Can sprinkle on everything if you really wanted to.
-Energy: The health pioneer Paul Bragg did an experiment an endurance hike with friends. They divided up into a Chia-eating group and another group, who ate whatever they wanted. The group eating only Chia seeds finished the hike four hours, twenty-seven minutes before the others, most of whom didn't even finish at all.
-Substitute: Use the Chia gel for baking!
-Clean: It helps to cleanse the intestines.
-Weight-loss: The combination of feeling fuller and cleansing the body equals a slimmer waistline.
So this magic food helps to keep your body in tip top condition, keeps you looking young, vibrant and feeling your best!

Dark chocolate is the best and has antioxidants, which I have discussed before.   Enjoying 3 oz with a few almonds mixed in is great. This amount of chocolate is just the right amount.   Dark chocolate has many known benefits, but it also can help put your body in the mood, and help you lose weight. If you can't do straight-up dark, do Chuaho chocolate pods. They are 60% dark. You may find more information on their website, www.chuaochocolatier.com.

Salty and fried foods can make skin and hair look dull and it can make it difficult to achieve orgasm. (They can affect you so negatively that you do not have an orgasm. No joke!!! So try to stay away from salty and fried food. You want your plate to be colorful with as many colors as the rainbow. (Talk about eating happy!)

Here is an example of what I think your plate should look like:

(I drew this example...I'm not an artist, as you can tell.)

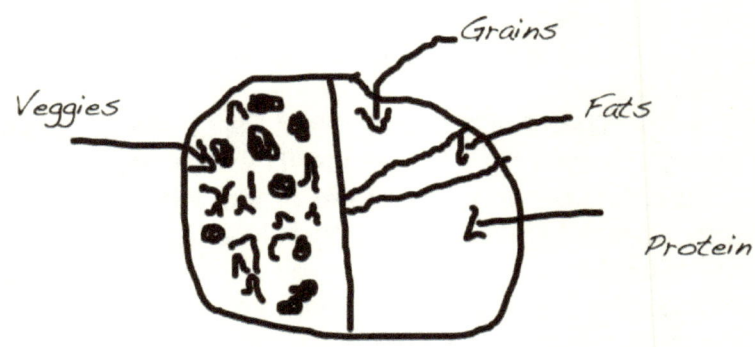

Some foods that may be harmful to your sexual body
    In particular, dairy. This is just my opinion, but here is some of the research that I found. Don't go by what I say, though, make your own educated decision. Some people very close to me will never give up dairy. Every now and again, I cook with it. How else am I to make delicious whipped cream? The following are not meant to scare you, or deter you from eating dairy. I have included them to make you think about what you put in your body just because someone else told you it was healthy.

-After the age of three the human body stops being able to break down dairy products.

-The African Bantu consume about 350mg of calcium per day. They rarely have a broken bone or lose their teeth and there is no calcium deficiency.

-Americans consume about 1000mg of calcium per day

-Native Eskimos consume about 2000mg of calcium per day and have the highest rate for Osteoporosis in the world!

Here are some of my favorite alternatives to dairy
-Soy Milk, Soy Cheese, Soy Yogurt, Soy Ice Cream (Soy may lower men's libidos. I have also found that I tend to gain a pound or two eating soy. Everyone is different. Test and   experience for yourself.)
-Rice Milk, Rice Cheese (not as "plastic" as it used to be!)
-Almond Milk (Huge fan!)
-Hemp Milk, Hemp Cheese

      If you follow this diet you will have no problem finding balance within your body. These foods help to naturally shed weight, will benefit your sex life, and make you glow with health and happiness. If you stick to fewer processed foods, eat fresh fruits and veggies, you will find your body improves, and your sex life will, too. Everything within your body is connected. If you are missing one part of the puzzle, it cannot be complete. Eating right is a special puzzle piece that people often forget about and neglect. Start today by putting the right foods in your body. When your body is in balance everything else finds its balance, as well. Within no time you'll be feeling better about yourself, and enjoying life to the fullest.

"In my end is my beginning."

-T.S. Eliot

When I truly listen to my body and supply its needs, I find myself easily being happy, fit and feeling good about how I look. The human mind is the best machine ever invented. Sure, there are a few glitches here and there. From time to time, faulty software has been downloaded. Just download a software upgrade and you'll be back in business. When I listen to my body, I know I will have an upset stomach when I drink milk. My body becomes bloated when I eat tofu, and my knees hate lunges. What should I do? I should adapt. It's survival. I try to avoid milk and tofu. When I work out I find an exercise that targets those muscle groups that my body will be able to handle in substitute for the lunges. So, listen to your body. Sometimes what you need to change is as simple as one thing. Other times it's a complete life, or physical, overhaul.

Having a healthy, fit body means more than a healthy diet and exercise. The largest component to a healthy body is the one that most people tend to forget about, or disregard, the mind. If you don't have a healthy mind and spirit you're doing your overall body's health a disservice. You'll over- or under-work your body and mind if these two aspects of your Self are not in balance.

I don't like the idea of depriving myself. I understand religious reasoning, (i.e.: Giving something up for your spiritual well-being.) Fasting can clear your mind of "wants," or at the very least, help you to feel closer to God. Most of us earthlings too often deprive ourselves of something, then turn around and act out in destructive ways. What is happiness? What is beautiful? The two are, more often than not, connected.

Outer beauty is fleeting and takes place in a finite period of time. Real beauty is within and lasting. Why do we want to be beautiful? The answer (that I have come up with) boils down to finding a suitable mate. My theory is, it is our human instinct to find a mate and reproduce. Nowadays, what is really beautiful has been skewed by the media and Hollywood. These two powerful forces have embedded little ticking time bombs into our brains. They make us believe that to be beautiful means to be thin, have large breasts, perfect skin, no rolls of fat, wrinkles, or visible cellulite, and do this all while wearing the latest fashion! The end result is, if you follow the mainstream beliefs, everyone will end up looking and being exactly the same. We would resemble little cookie-cutter people walking down the street, single file.

When I was young and fretting about an outfit, or worried about what others might think of me, my mother used to say, "What's the worst thing that could happen? They might laugh at you? Then you made someone happy. If you can live with the worst thing that could happen, go for it! It doesn't matter what other people think."

Our current society doesn't like change and it certainly doesn't embrace the term "different." Imagine a world where you could be truly yourself and accepted for it. Today, to receive this sort of acceptance, someone has to be in love with you. I long for the day when people will feel free to wear what makes them feel good and not to care if lines are starting to show up on their faces. I have observed that the older someone is the more they tend to come into their own. They no longer want to keep up with the Joneses, and are more secure with the way they look. Every day is a struggle for me. Some days I feel wonderful, beautiful and witty! Within 24 hours, I could discover none of my clothes fit me, I want to hide my face, and somehow, when I open my mouth all that seems to come out is gibberish and nonsense!

It is my belief that when we enter this world, we have a job to do, or a life purpose, which can bring us (and others) great joy. It is also my belief that we know or have an idea of what our life purpose is when we our young. If you look back to your childhood, what were your interests, your talents? Try to remember, what was the main thing that brought joy to your life? Speaking for myself, I had many interests. I loved to write plays and music, sing, dance and I was always trying to invent something new. Even with all of these interests, there was one topic that stood out to me, Love.

It wasn't really an interest as much as it was a calling in Life. I knew deep down in my soul that I wanted it, even though I didn't really know what it was, or what it entailed. We are all born with a certain, God-given purpose, and there are certain things that we need to achieve within our lifetime. Maybe you were born to be the mother of an activist, or maybe you were born to travel the world. Everyone's purpose is just as important as the next person's. Being the President of the United States is just as important as being a housewife in Omaha, Nebraska. Why? Because everything we do in this world within our own lifetime has an effect on the future, and on someone else. So, to say one person is more important than another is just not the truth. Sometimes, even the way we die is our purpose in life. Tragic accidents happen all the time. Sometimes, even though a tragedy did happen, it results in changes to laws, there will be more safety precautions taken, and lives will be ultimately being saved.

Figure out what brings you joy in this world. We are merely a flicker of light, and our life here is precious and no monetary value may be placed on it.   Time is short, but always high in demand. We always want more of it, and we always think we have another day.

Grateful

"Promise me you'll always remember: You're braver than you believe, and stronger than you seem, and smarter than you think."

-Christopher Robin to Pooh, A.A. Milne

I am so very grateful that I was able to write this book. It has been a dream of mine for years and now it's a reality. I have been lucky enough to have the love and support of my family and friends. In return, I am very lucky to have a family I love and cherish. They are my world. I am also very fortunate to have friends who I would do almost anything for, and who would do the same for me. Never in my life have I felt as loved as I do at this very moment. I am surrounded by love. Because I am loved and supported, I am able to do anything, especially in my efforts to keep my body healthy.

Sometimes we search and search for something only to realize we already have everything we need. If we would open up our eyes to all the possibilities and the wonderful things that happen to us every day, I am positive that each and every day would be the best day ever. I used to think otherwise: I used to believe that there was only one person who could "complete" you. Now, many years later, I have come to the realization that my life is already fulfilling and full of love. Every day there is Joy waiting for me!

You don't have to be in a relationship to receive the benefits that love can provide. You just need to love yourself and have the love of friends. True friends inspire us, they support us, and make us feel better about ourselves. I am lucky to have friends all over the world. I have lived in many places, and along this jumbled path, I have made some amazing folks who have become lifelong friends. These friends have shown me real love, and shown me how to love. Love is bountiful. It should be part of your work-out plan to spend time with your best friends! The laughter alone is a workout and a calorie burner. So, fall in love with your friends and family again!

Thank you to my mother Catherine and my little sister Ada for helping me with the editing of this book. You help to mask my borderline illiteracy! Thank you to Bill Hoenk Photography for capturing the book photo. You make me look as good as I feel and I thank you for that. Thank you to my family and friends who have been so supportive of me and this venture. I couldn't have written this book, nor been so successful, without your love and support. Being loved for who you are makes life easy and worth living. A sincere heartfelt thank you to anyone who has ever inspired me, broken my heart, or made me laugh. I thank you for the experiences, good and bad.

In no particular order (and I apologize if I inadvertently omit anyone) thank you to: Catherine Flanagan Stover, John H. Stover, AdaRuth Stover, Perry Stover Wotring, Cora Stover, Ada Stover, Dorothy Locke, Jen Hanlon, Donna and Kevin Hanlon, Lynn and Frank Cushing, Ruth Ann Flanagan, Liz Flanagan, Dan and Janet Flanagan, Erin Flanagan Roberts, Reyna Kerzic, Kelly Miller, Catherine Tran, Julie Darby, Amanda Morgan, Janine Mauldin, Meri Lepore, Sabrina Clark, Kay, Jessica Handley, Don Wotring, Bill Hoenk, Eli Stover, Isaiah Stover, and Brett Morneau.

Quick Reference Guide

-Drink Wine

-Spoonful of Olive Oil when hungry, a spoonful in the morning and before you go to bed

-3 oz of Dark Chocolate

-Eat a couple of nuts before a meal

-Eat good fats like avocados

-Chia seeds - Two spoonfuls a day

-Eat lots of fruits and veggies especially pineapples, oranges, bananas and green veggies

-Drink Green Tea - 5 cups a day

-Say "I love you"

-Eat "clean" foods, nothing processed

-Skip the "junk" unless you make it yourself

-Enjoy sex with a partner, or by yourself.

-Laugh all day, everyday

-And, above all, LOVE!

About the Author

Dorothy Stover is a good girl with mischievous tendencies (nicknamed "Naughty-Dottie" at a very young age by her parental units.)

She has been in love with life for years now, and doesn't expect that to change any time soon.

She loves active-and-inactive-activities.

She listens to her Mother: "Intelligent people are never bored."

At times, Dorothy had a difficult relationship. With herself. But, making the decision to be a "victor" instead of a "victim" has allowed her to build a solid, healthy relationship. With herself. What has evolved is a committed relationship (with herself) constructed on a foundation of friendship, trust, excitement, hope, and always LOVE!

Follow her blog a www.lazypersonaltraining.com or find her on Twitter with the rest of the mainstream celebrities at @Doro727.

Amazing Love Diet

Dorothy D Stover

USA

Amazing Love Diet

I dedicate this book to the women in my life, especially my Mother. You have shown me real beauty, and what it means to love yourself for who you really are.

Foreword

This is the second edition of Amazing Love Diet. I pulled the first edition off the shelves due to the sexual content and my amazing spelling and grammatical errors. (Can you believe it? I even spelled grammar wrong!)

Obviously spelling is not my forte. I think of myself as an ideas girl. I am usually 'in my head,' thinking about whatever is going on up there. I love to write, which is why that's what I do. Am I any good at it? Perhaps. Is the content in this book information that I happen to be the only one who understands, or knows? No. This book is a compilation of what I have learned in (what some consider) my few, short years on this planet. I am still learning and discovering. I am an observer, and I have a great memory for events. This has enabled me to tell you what I know. At least, a small portion of what I have learned. A girl has to save some secrets for herself!

When I first set out to write this book I was excited and thrilled. I thought about writing this book for many years before I ever set my fingers to the keyboard. As time went on and I was engrossed in writing, I realized how much of myself I was actually putting into this book. The thought that people would know so much about me was, and is, so scary. That was the primary reason for my taking so long to complete the first edition, and why it has taken me so long to complete this second edition. It's as if I am walking down the street completely naked and exposed. There are certainly moments when I love being in my invisible bikini and strutting my stuff like the proud lioness that I am. Then there are those frightening moments when I realize I am the only one without cover, and I begin to rethink my courage to stand apart from the crowd.

Once I started this book there was no other option but to finish. I have completed this journey of writing Amazing Love Diet. I am proud of myself for taking a risk and putting myself out there. I hope you enjoy this glimpse into my world. I hope you are entertained, and perhaps learn something you didn't know before. I hope that you are inspired. Inspired to love. Inspired to live life to the fullest. Inspired to branch out and take your own risks in life. The reward could be great. You'll only know if you try. Thank you so much for your support, and as always Much Love to You.

PS. Sorry to anyone who was really looking forward to the Sexercises. I plan on releasing that information in more detail in a future publication.

The Beginning - My Story

"All our knowledge has its origins in our perceptions."
-Leonardo da Vinci

Within this book you will find the secrets to a beautiful body. Achieving this is easier than you might think. I have put in years of research, time and experience through my travels to find the story of how love can transform your body and your mind. I am living proof that the effort one puts into love can yield a greater reward.

For you to truly understand this book, you need to know where I am coming from. I have a few stories about how I became me! My first story will be about my body and mind. The second is a story about love. The third story is a mystery! (This trifecta ultimately revealed me to ME!) This is the foundation. Later in the book, I will share with you my secrets to love and achieving a beautiful body. Love, and what we put in our bodies, plays a major role in achieving this.

My Body and Mind

There are many different aspects to my body. I am tall. I am never the same weight two days in a row. I wear glasses. I have wavy, unruly hair. I have small feet. I am awkward. I have an hourglass figure. I have a pointy nose. I have small hands. I have hazel eyes. I have an "innie" for a bellybutton. My voice resembles that of a five year old. I am a bad speller. I love to eat. I love to drink Champagne. My grammar is wretched. I can't do a cartwheel. Open water calms me down. I am obsessive. I am lazy. I am energetic. (I am contradictory!) I have long legs. I am territorial. I can be weird. I talk too much. I am happy. I love.

I didn't know anything was wrong with me until I started grade school. Children have a spectacular way of singling someone out. First of all, I was smaller in stature than the other kids and extremely thin. I wore glasses and marched (frenziedly) to a different drummer. This combination isn't a good one for being popular. It was difficult even getting by without someone taking the time to notice me in a negative light. This all added up to many days coming home crying to my Mother who always knew exactly what to say to make me feel better. "You tell those kids that if they don't leave you alone, I'm going to come down there and hang them up by their toes."

My mother is a powerhouse standing at about 5' 2" with flaming red hair. She may be little in size but you would never want to mess around with her, or make my mother angry. You would soon come to the realization that doing so was a bad idea. So, backed with my mother's strong spirit, I held my head higher and started to fight my own battles. Sometimes with my fists, sometimes with words. Soon children in grade school did stop picking on me, but they would eventually pick on someone else. In turn, I found myself fighting for others who, like me, were afraid to speak up, or defend themselves against the terrifying eight year olds.

As time went on I became more awkward and my height shot up to make me one of the tallest in the class. This really didn't help my case as I was still super-thin and had my bottle cap glasses. Children came up with very clever names like "Spider Dot" or "Dotty-long-legs." My mother gave me solid, wonderful, wise advise. She would say to me, "Just ignore them. Nothing makes someone angrier than when you ignore them." I found this statement to be nonsensical at the time. I wanted to take my abnormally small hands and ring their little necks. I thought this would be the best way to shut them up. Eventually, after much consideration, I took my mother's advice and just ignored the kids. I learned to develop a thick skin where name-calling was concerned.

Our growing-up years lay the foundation for who we are, and who we will become. Our parents can only do their best and what they consider is right for their children.

Society can also play a major role in how we act and feel about ourselves. It's sad, but it's the truth. We all have short comings that people are more than happy to expose and profit over, all while overlooking their own. Every event, every experience, every person who touches our lives, even the ones that seem insignificant at the time, all shape who we are.

When I was 19 years old, I became very sick. I was taking roughly 23 supplements daily and was only allowed to eat certain foods. The main food items I had to cut out were dairy, wheat, yeast and gluten. At the time there weren't as many healthy food choices on the shelves in the grocery that met my requirements. Even at health food stores it was hard to find food that met all of my needs. Sure, there were some items available, but not the selection that we know today. Now you may walk into any common grocery store and find something that will conform to most dietary restrictions, and it will taste good. Almost like the real thing! Almost.

The lowest point in my food life was right after I was diagnosed. My mother took me to the grocery store to gather all my new "eats." Moms in general know how to make everything better, and my mother in particular has quite the talent for it. She made me feel special and cared for. Unfortunately, that all disappeared when I was sitting in my dorm room craving a grilled cheese sandwich, one of my favorite comfort foods. I wasn't going to let this "bump in the road" stop me from enjoying life, and I was determined to make my own grilled cheese sandwich.

I took out my wheat free, yeast free, gluten free, (taste free) cardboard bread and added my "plastic-looking" rice cheese to the center of the two slices. I took out my toaster oven. (Now, I know you're not supposed to have a toaster oven in your dorm room. I had special permission because of my circumstances.) I placed my little makeshift grilled cheese in the toaster oven. I continued to watch my grilled cheese with anticipation. I was so excited for it to be done, and couldn't wait to sink my teeth into something yummy and gooey. As I stared through the glass at my sandwich, my smile started to turn upside down. I watched as the edges of the bread turned upwards away from the rice "plastic-looking" cheese. Then the buzzer went off. With a positive attitude and a grumbling stomach I took out my little sandwich and had my first bite. This was followed by tears streaming down my face. I sat in my dorm room crying and couldn't stop crying and continued to eat my grilled cheese. To my surprise and disappointment my sandwich didn't have any of the yummy, comforting gooeyness that I was craving. Instead, this grilled cheese tasted just like it looked: two pieces of cardboard with a slice of plastic in the middle. That was my lowest moment in my food life. (I would learn a valuable lesson that day: never cry while you're eating.)

Now, I had to change my diet to save my life and to get better. Eventually, I did get my health back and once I was healed, I was able to add certain foods back into my diet. You may not be in such a predicament, but still your life and food situation is just as critical as mine was. You need to get yourself to the healthy point, and then you can start adding more foods into your diet. Our bodies are always in need of balance.

On to my second story about Love.

Love

Growing up, I was obsessed with love and finding my soul mate. I was a true romantic. As a child, all I wanted to do was get married to someone who I loved madly, and who loved me back in the same way. We would make a family together! For many years I carried around a tiny toy baby. I loved this baby more than anything and truly believed I was this toy baby's mother.

Amazing Love Diet

Over time, my excessive love for this baby would result in a weakening of the doll's fabric "skin." A tear in a leg, an arm, or her torso would appear, here or there, and would have to be duct-taped. Within a few years the baby had a duct-tape diaper and body suit. The painted on eyes started to fade and my baby looked more like a grey ball of duck tape than the cute snuggly baby that it once had been. That is a part of love, isn't it? The original thing we started off with changes shape, becoming something completely different, almost to the point of being unrecognizable. The only thing that recognizes it is your heart's eye. Your heart has vision better than 20/20.

My one was goal in life at a very early age was to fall in love. When I learned what people did with each other when they were in love (sex), well, this just fueled my drive for love and my search for my soul mate. I had the scenario all planned in my head. I would lose my virginity to the person I was going to be with for the rest of my life. We would have a beautiful night of sweet kisses, caressing each other's bodies, and intense, soulful eye contact. This was my dream and I would wait until the day I found this special person. We would give ourselves, our whole selves, to each other. It was a sweet dream, one I held onto, even to this day.

The years passed, my body and I changed, but I never abandoned my ultimate goal. Of course, I felt pressure in middle school and high school to find someone to lose my virginity to. My friends all had boyfriends. And me? Well, it was a rarity for any boy to look at me since I towered over most of them and resembled a two-by-four board with Coke-bottle glasses and had braces to boot. I still put pressure on myself, thinking, he's just around the corner. You just have to wait a little bit longer.

As time went on I thought if I was going to find someone, I'd better look more like my friends. They all had shapely bodies and wore more revealing clothing. I come from a very strict Catholic family with conservative parents. At least where fashion was concerned. Wearing a skirt, shorts or a shirt that was too short was forbidden. I remember coming down all dressed for school one morning, and started making my breakfast. I reached up to the top cabinet for my favorite cereal – Cinnamon Toast Crunch. My Mother yelped, "Is that your belly? Go change your shirt." My shirt was (maybe) showing an inch of my skin while my hands were above my head. When my parents would stop me, abruptly, from leaving the house in whatever get up I may have been wearing, all I could think about was, "I'll never find a boyfriend. And I'll never have sex." I would later go on to find out it truly doesn't matter what someone may look like or what someone may wear. If you want sex, more than likely someone will be ready and willing to oblige you. I have also discovered that there is someone for everyone. If you have a big nose, I bet there is someone out there who is going to think your nose is the sexiest nose on the planet. Best advice: Just be who you are, someone will fall in love with the genuine you.

Fashion-wise growing up, I was a bit of a dud. My parents had less than no interest in buying me clothes that were fashionable, like the other girls my age. They didn't want me dressing too "mature" for my age, and with good reason. There are some creepy, disturbed people in this world who prey upon young girls.

So, afflicted with conservative parents, a body that looked like a very long stick with glasses, and no fashion sense, in my own eyes I was doomed to never finding my soul mate. It was so rare that any guy, besides those over 40, would find me attractive. Soon, I found myself not believing the guy if he did like me.

I once read a book that said that before we come on to this earth we choose our families. Evidently, before we get here, somehow we know what we have to work on during our lifetime, and we know how long we will stay on this earth. I would say I am starting to agree with this statement. I have always believed we know what we're supposed to be when we grown up at a very young age. We know what impact we are going to make on the world by the time we're five. At least in my opinion we do. Perhaps our parents have a different vision for us than the one we have. This, too, is part of what will shape and mold who you become. For the most part, we already "know" what we are going to be, we just don't know the details of the journey.

As a child, I didn't know what "being in love" was, but I knew that was for me! I wanted to meet my soul mate and grow old together. When I graduated from high school my Mother gave me a present. It was some type of time capsule. It was just a box made out of cardboard that she found at some store like Borders or Barnes and Noble. I remember her presenting this gift to me. The "capsule" was actually a shiny, blue, rectangular box with a painted-on yellow ribbon across the front. I opened up the box like a box of Russell Stover chocolates to find multiple questionnaires with matching envelopes. I was supposed to hand each questionnaire to a friend or family member to fill out. I also had my own questionnaire to fill out. Once all the questionnaires were completed each person would seal their envelope and place it in the box. I would have to wait 10 years before being able to open each letter. Talk about anticipation!

Throughout those 10 years of waiting, I remember wondering what my family and friends would write about me. How did they see my future? Will I be a completely different person in 10 years, or will I be the same? Will everything that I want come true? Ten years did eventually pass. One day, out of the blue, I came upon the blue time capsule box. I was extremely nervous and apprehensive about what I was going to find inside. I opened each envelope with excitement and enthusiasm. It felt like

Christmas and each letter was a small gift for me to unwrap! Much to my surprise, the life that people thought I would be living was quite different than the reality. It was as different as the world I had thought for myself. My family, friends and I all thought that by age 28 or 29, I would be married with a family!

Little did I know back then, but it's a long road from where you think you should be and where you are. I have experienced more pain than I would want my worst enemy to go through. Still, with all the heartache and pain, I believe in love. I still believe in the good. I still hope. I have found the good through love of myself, travel, and love of others. Let me share with you what I've learned thus far on my journey in life. I   believe the love of ourselves is the greatest treasure we will ever behold.

The Journey to Love

"And think not you can direct the course of love, for love, if it finds you worthy, directs your course."
-Khalil Gibran

"To thine own self be true." I believe Shakespeare meant this line to mean, "Take care of yourself first." I also believe you shouldn't take this as an excuse to be selfish. Certainly though, you must secure your own oxygen mask before helping others secure theirs. What good are you to others if you are not 100%? This is a lesson I have learned over and over again. Take care of yourself, before taking care of others. The journey to Love is a journey to loving yourself. Loving yourself, in turn, allows you to have the body and the life that you need. (Notice how I didn't say want?) What we want, may not be and most likely is not, what we need. I would love to be 5'2" and 110 pounds. Guess what? That will never happen and I've accepted it. Love yourself for your unique self, eat well, and love every moment, even if you have pain in your heart.

I have often felt that life is beautiful. Almost perfect, the way things seem to work out. Even in my darkest moments I've tried to find the good. Eventually the good always finds a way back into my life. Those dark moments are the real moments in our lives that truly shape the person who we are and who we will become. It's those moments when we are staring at fear and pain that really make life worth living. If every day were perfect, you wouldn't actually know what perfect was. If you never had a bad day, you would never know what a good day feels like. So, when you do experience the bad in life, remember it. Learn from it. Heal from it, knowing that good is around the corner, waiting silently for you. I would care to wager, that once you've experience the bad, you hold on that much tighter to the good in life. Maybe even treasure it just a little more than when you did in your past. I know I have and do.

When I have bad days, weeks, months or even years, it gives me comfort to know that somewhere in my future there will be good again. The journey to love is rough terrain. There are ups and downs. There will be moments when you don't believe you are worth it and then there will be moments when you know you are.

In my experience, and what I have observed in my few years on this planet, is most people go through some sort of trauma. This acts as a trigger. This trigger may set you off on an unhealthy path. Maybe even a destructive path. This is just a mere distraction if you break down the trigger. Once you have discovered what your particular trigger is that set you on an unhealthy path, you will be empowered to change what you need to change to chart your course on to the smoother road to love.

How to discover your trigger:

For me, I tried to diligently keep track of how I feel, what I do when something upsets me. What I discovered was, when I am upset or in need of comfort I tend to turn to food. I have noticed that when I am unhappy, even if I am eating fairly well, I still gain weight. When I am happy in my life, somehow pounds just fall off and stay off. So, my greatest health secret is to be happy with myself and love myself...But that you already know.

To discover what may set you off on the wrong path listen to what happens to your mind, your body, and your spirit when something upsets you. What do you remember? Write everything down, even if it seems small and insignificant. It's sometimes the little things in our everyday that can make us upset and create a toxin in our system.

I know for me when a romantic relationship ends, it triggers a lot of my bad habits. I won't eat right. I won't take walks or be active in any way. I hit rock bottom every-time, until I am able to recognize that this is one of my triggers. Sure, I still grab a bag of BBQ chips and a pint of Ben and Jerry's Half Baked but I don't hate myself for it. I recognize that it's a temporary fix. Then I move on and do the work to move on from the relationship and get myself back to 100% both in body, mind and spirit.

I have found in my past that even when I was in a relationship I was truly single. So I learned to love myself. If I didn't love who I was then how could someone love me if I didn't love myself? I think this is simple logic, just not as simple to accomplish. I have often found myself comparing my mind and body to others. When I should accept myself for who I am, all of my talents and all of my beauties.

Here is a Self-Love Exercise, Beautiful Body, which I have taught others. This exercise will help you to fall in love with your own body. This may take time and repetitive repetitions to gain the full benefits. Anything worth achieving does require effort and work on each individual.

I suggest you start off by looking at your naked body in the mirror. Be your best friend. Best friends will always tell you that you look beautiful and bring your spirits up. So what would your friends say to you? Start off by pointing out the positive in yourself. What is your favorite feature? Maybe it's your eyes, butt, and legs or maybe it's your chest, arms and feet. Whatever the case may be, it's all you and you should enjoy it. No one else on this planet is put together quite like you, and that's something to be proud of.

Over time, the effort you made in appreciating yourself, you will find that you are happier with you and your body. You will be amazed what a happier you will do for your spirit and your health. You may even find yourself accepting those dimples on your tummy or cellulite on your thighs. Start today, take off all your clothes and bask in the glory of you and your body.

THE AMAZING LOVE DIET IS BORN

"Take care of your body. It's the only place you have to live."

- Jim Rohn

Family Girl

I am very close to my family. They are my best friends and biggest supporters. I come from a large, loud family, sort of like the one in My Big Fat Greek Wedding. There are always a dozen simultaneous conversations going on, everyone talking to the point you can hardly hear. And, there is always amazing food! I would much rather stay home and watch a movie with my family and eat and eat and eat than to go out "drinking until I can't see any more!"

I just love my family. We laugh all the time, we fight like crazy people, and we always have something delicious for dinner and dessert. I am one of six children. I have two older brothers who would steal the food off my fork. I have an older sister who showed me "the ropes," and told me what to do. I have two younger sisters who I bossed around and tried to make my personal "slaves." Growing up in a big family you gain an enhanced appreciation for food, especially in sufficient quantities. My friends found it incredible how fast I could eat and how I didn't say a word during a meal. The reason for this was, with six kids (and two big older brothers) if you didn't eat fast, you didn't eat. The food was so good and there were plenty of mouths that wanted to eat it. If I wanted seconds, and didn't want my big brothers to eat the food right off my fork, I had to move quickly. So, my food obsession started with my family and my mother's cooking. There is nothing like my mother's cooking. Dessert, for sure, is her specialty and I couldn't get enough.

My experience filling a void with food was something I discovered was while I was going to school in

Florida. I was happy living there. I had great friends, I loved my school, and it was sunny almost all of the time. Coming from the Northeast, that sunny weather was a blessing. I was used to freezing winters, a rainy spring, sticky summers and a grey fall. The problem with Florida was, I discovered, I missed my family. I stuffed my mouth with food. I wasn't listening to my body and its dietary needs. I wasn't eating because I was hungry, and I wasn't eating food that was good for me, I was eating because I missed my family. I gained about 30 pounds of "missing." No one really noticed because I am 5'10" so I was able to hide it well. I went on eating like this for quite some time, just to comfort myself and to attempt to fill the void. Well, at least I thought I did. I once asked my one of my brothers if he could tell I gained weight. His reply, "A little." I had developed this unhappy food habit, and my quality of life went down. I also started seeing a real jerk of a guy who didn't care about my needs, just his own. Funny when you're not 100% you attract others who are not 100%. For a half a year, I wallowed in this mess. Then, BOOM! I finally ended it with the guy and decided I was going to look and feel amazing!

I first started with a list of what I wanted and formed my goals were. I wanted a tip-top shape of a peach, aka my vagina. I wanted my head of hair to grow faster and stronger. I wanted my skin to glow. I researched and found the foods that would facilitate these results. That list of helpful food was all I ate during this time of my recreating myself. I also wasn't dating anyone at this time and kept to my normal routine of pleasuring myself. Honestly, sometimes it isn't worth the trouble of being in a relationship. Especially, if your partner is selfish in bed and in life. What is the point of being with them? So you don't feel alone? You're alone, trust me. You just have someone around to remind you of how alone you are. Once I realized this and kept to the diet, I found that within a month or two I had completely changed my body. My skin, hair, and peach were glowing! (And, I had six-pack abs.) I lost 25 pounds in just a few short months and kept it off.

The birth of the Amazing Love Diet! With more research, I found you can eat for great sex. This great sex doesn't have to be with a partner. I know this because I'm the type of girl who wants a monogamous relationship. I haven't had many partners for fear of what my Mother had always told me: "You will become attached to every person you sleep with." This statement has always scared "the real" into me. Much like what you might say to a child when they've swallowed their chewing gum, "Don't swallow that gum. It will stay in your belly forever!" With this fear of inappropriate attachments, I became the type of girl who could please herself sexually. Practice makes perfect, or so I've heard.

I wasn't going to sleep with just anyone. Even now, as then, there are rigid pre-qualifications: I have to be in love with him, or have a crazy-strong physical attraction to that person. Either one is not easy for me. (Probably why I found myself flying solo!) I have to know he's in it for the long haul, and can handle me. I'm a lot to handle behind closed doors, and not for the faint of heart. My best 48 hours with a guy, we didn't eat any food whatsoever, and I think we got a total of two hours of sleep. When we did come up for air, we ordered take out. So you can see, you have to keep up! I'm the Energizer Bunny. Sometimes sex is "food" for me, and sometimes food is "sex for me." I'm in a constant balancing act.

When I was 12 years old, I read an article on exercise and orgasms, and how they coincide. The article listed 30 different forms of exercise. Some examples: Yoga, Pilates, Running, Walking, Horse Back Riding, Swimming, etc. Along with this helpful list was a poll asking 100 women from each different exercise group about certain aspects of their lifestyle, concentrating on fitness, health and their sex lives. The data was gathered and quantified. The article then listed each exercise along with the percentage of women who experienced frequent orgasms within each grouping. The bottom of this list was running or jogging. Only 23% of women who ran for exercise had frequent orgasms. The top of the list was Pilates, rating at 99% of women having frequent orgasms. I bought a Pilates DVD the very next day.

I should disclose (and my parents will be relieved to learn) that I was not sexually active at 12 years old. Far, far from it. I have had an obsession with sex all my life, even before I really knew what the birds and the bees were. I have always been a fervent reader, gleaning as much information as possible on the subject. You may consider this your gain, as I will pass on my knowledge to you! (Well, as much knowledge as someone can gain at my age and experience.)

As you may have guessed, I am obsessed with sex, always have been, and always will be. I wanted to be sure that when the day finally came for me to be "a woman," I was going to be the best in bed. So, I would kiss every wall in my house, or practice on my hand with the hope that, one day, it would be a real honest-to-goodness tall, dark and handsome man or woman. I was open to all possibilities. The kissing obsessions soon lead to everything to do with sex. I was a sponge, taking all this information in. Now that I am older, I have been able to put my studying into use. In bed I am what they call a "pleaser." I want to make sure my partner is satisfied. I learn what they like, what they really like, and I do it. For me, my pleasure comes from pleasing someone else. I also know how to please myself. I've been practicing since I was about three or four years old. Back then, I didn't know what I was doing, but it felt great. I realized when I got older what was going on. I'll get into that later, because it's important to know how to please yourself.

Amazing Love Diet

To repeat, food and sex have always been my passions. I believe, because I was always so obsessed with sex and my body, it has given me an advantage sexually. When I finally learned to read, I would gather all the information I could on sex. My primary goal was to be the best in bed for my future spouse. Naturally, all this information wouldn't be in play until many, many years down the road, but I wanted to be ready for it, nevertheless!

In my years on this planet, I have found that health and a beautiful body begin within your mind. When you really want something, you are willing to invest whatever it takes to acquire your desire. Whether it be shopping for just the right dress for an up-coming party, or finding the perfect birthday present for that special someone. The desire and the want all start in your mind. The compulsion to get that "perfect something" all starts within you.

When I was a little girl, I told my mother at our dinner table that the way to get a boy to love you was to bat your eyelashes. She just smiled and said, "Oh! Is that how it's done?" I have always had an obsession with love. In some circles they would call it "a passion". For me, it truly was.

Being in love is one of the most amazing feelings you can ever experience. I had a great love, and let me tell you, he could do no wrong in my eyes. Every day I would run to that door to greet the man I couldn't stand to be without. I was much like a puppy. He could have come home and said, "Well it's done. I've killed everyone, and I mean everyone! We are the only two people left." In my sick way, I would have thought, How romantic. I have the best guy ever! Granted, that is an amazing love, but amazingly messed up. Happily, that kind of "love" has faded, and the journey continues.

Amazing Love Diet

For as long as I can remember, my Mother has given me self-help books. They are mainly in regard to love and relationships. It started off with the best seller, Are you there God? It's Me, Margaret. This original self-help book relates a young girl's trials of loving her new body and God. After this little gem, my Mother was on a roll, gifting me with only the crème de la crème of self help books. Books like, He's Just Not That into You, and Steve Harvey's book, Act like a Lady, Think like a Man. Recently, I came to the edge when she handed me her latest find, How to Know If He's Going to Marry You In 30 Days or Less. Now, all things being considered, I'm a lucky girl. I've had a few marriage proposals, some of them serious, some of them not. I'm a girl who loves love and would someday like to have a spouse and a few ankle biters of my own. I believe I would thrive as a wife and mother. It could very well be my calling in life.

I have always been obsessed with finding the right partner to spend the rest of my life with. My Mother and I have a strong bond, and certainly this obsession has played a role in our bond. Over the years, I've had some bad luck in the love department, but I've had some magical moments, too. Falling in love is a beautiful thing. Falling out of love is a process we all have to go through to grow. "Grow with love," as they say.

There was one guy I really thought was going to make my dreams a reality. Except the reality was, I wasn't ready to get married! I had many items on my "Things to Do Before 'I Do' " list. This was a considerably long list, consisting of all my wants and desires. I wanted to travel by myself. I wanted to crash a wedding. I wanted a small career success, and many, many more fun things I just couldn't do if I were married. My desire to be in a healthy, happy marriage notwithstanding, I wasn't quite ready to be in wedded bliss, especially with this list looming over me. Recently I realized that I don't have anything left to do on my list! Maybe, just maybe, I'm ready now that I've completed all the "To Do's?"

My mother has seen me struggle over the years within my romantic relationships, as well as with my weight. She is always trying to help me find my way. This is what makes her a great mother. She wants only the best for me. That was the reason she was constantly handing me the self-help books. It was just another way of trying to help me find my way. I understand where my mother was coming from. It was from a place of love. She only wanted me to be happy. She's seen my heart get broken, but she also wants grand-babies before she's in diapers herself. She knows I've always wanted children, and that playing 'house' was my favorite game as a little girl.

What is this need to see the ones we love paired off, and married? My older sister married when she was twenty-five years old. I was twenty-three at the time. My grandmother said to me the week of the wedding, right after I had broken up with my boyfriend, "Don't worry dear. Twenty-three isn't considered an old maid anymore." I was in shock. Happily, she followed up her comment with, "You're beautiful. You'll have no trouble finding a husband." Thanks, Granny! (I think?)

With so many "self-help" books out there I wanted to write something that was really about "helping you." I love the term, "self -help book." This terminology openly states and affirms that all you need is your self. You are the only person who can help yourself. Sure, others can inspire you and guide you on your path, but when it comes down to the work, you are the only person for the job. You don't need to be anything more than who you are. My goal is for women to feel beautiful about themselves, and to have great sex! That's all I want for them. This sex can be by yourself, or with a partner. I don't want you to count calories, or to worry about if you eat this or that, or berating yourself if you fall off the wagon. Those activities only bring you down. Truthfully, that is no way to live and enjoy life. To me, that is what I live for. I want to enjoy this life. Eat the foods I want, kiss the people I want and bask in how glorious it all was, and is. There are only a few people in this world who are truly happy counting calories. Doctors have a term for those people so afflicted: they are "suffering from" an eating disorder. No offense, but it's true. I am my happiest when I'm around friends and family, enjoying my favorite foods, laughing, and having a glass of very good wine. To me, that's what is worth living for (...and of course great sex!)

The key to a great sex life is confidence and knowing your body. Confidence comes from feeling good about yourself. With this way of life, you will feel better about yourself. You will, in turn, learn things about your body you never knew, or didn't want to admit. You might end up losing 10, 20, 30, or more pounds, but that is not the end goal. That is a bonus. The end goal is to feel beautiful and to have a great time with or without someone behind closed doors. And come on; let's face it that would mean a happy life, even if you couldn't lose those last few pounds.

I will tell you this: our bodies were made for sex. In fact we are sex machines. You may laugh, thinking that I'm crazy, but let's think about it. When you are having sex, your body releases so many happy chemicals! We are the only species on this planet that really enjoys sexual intercourse. We have sex for many different reasons, not just to make babies. We have sex to fall asleep. An orgasm is more powerful than a sleeping pill. We have sex because we are bored. (There don't seem to be any shows we like on the television, and we don't feel like reading a book.) We have sex because we just saw Ocean's 11, and there is enough visual beefcake for a woman to be satisfied for months. Variety is the spice of life. I've heard that some people have sex to keep their significant others from bothering them about last month's credit card bill. This is a morally "grey area," but the reality is their significant other stopped complaining about the bill, didn't they?

Women have sex for many reasons. Perhaps you already knew this, but are you enjoying your sex life? Do you like your body? Could there be improvements? I'm sure every woman answers differently. The truth is you're reading this because you are curious. At some point in every woman's sex life, things can take a downhill turn. (That's if you had an uphill to begin with.) 30% of women have never reached an orgasm. Let me repeat this because this just shouldn't be the case. 30% of women have never had an orgasm! The point of this book is to get you back up the hill or for you 30% out there who need to, to start climbing and reach the top of the orgasm mountain! When your body is in tip-top shape the body takes over and does its thing, just like a well oiled machine. And, when I say tip-top shape I'm not talking "bikini model." I am almost positive that they are not eating right to have an orgasm. You need certain things for your body to be well-oiled, but I will get into that later.

Sex: Whether by yourself or with a partner, this is an important part of looking and feeling amazing. Intercourse improves circulation, breaks up fatty tissue in your body, and improves your immune system function.

Over the years, I have learned that it doesn't matter what you say to try to talk someone out of something when they really want it, or desire it. They will, more than likely, still go after the guy who treats them like dirt, or drink a bottle of wine all by themselves at dinner. Neither of these habits is good for them, and the short and long-term effects can be brutal. No, there is nothing you can do for this friend until they are ready to listen.

Amazing Love Diet

So, until you are ready to listen to me, put down this book because nothing I will say will have any meaning to you. But, if you are ready to listen, you will find your world will change. Maybe not your whole universe, but parts of you will grow and develop into the person who you know you can be. We are always changing as people. Sure, there are parts of us that stay the same, but I bet if you give it enough time and attention, those parts will change as well. For example, as a child I hated tomatoes and mayonnaise. I didn't want tomatoes on my salad or in a sandwich. I just couldn't stand it. Now, as an adult I love them, and they are an important part of my diet and well-being. Still, when it comes to mayonnaise, I still don't like it. I can tolerate it if I'm at a summer barbecue (which always seems laden with mayonnaise items!) So, you see, people can change. It's just a matter of when, where, and why.

Back to your mind and your beautiful body! When you are feeling true to yourself, the pounds will start to fall off. It's a combination of you being you, and not caring what people think. When you worry about what people think, you tend not to eat right. I know this because I've been through it. I spent many years trying to change my concern that people's opinions about me matter to me. They just don't, in the long run. Their judgment of you is just that. Judgment, and who are they to judge? I have discovered that people are usually too wrapped up in themselves and how things will affect them, than how they will affect you.

When I was 16, I was sexually assaulted. It was a brutal attack, not just to my body, but to some of the hopes and dreams of what a girl wants to experience when she makes love for the first time. Obviously, this wasn't making love. Love and kindness were nowhere to be seen on that night. Still, what happened happened. I've traveled my path and have grown every step of the way. I would hit bumps along the road, and I would struggle to get over them. One bump in particular was with my body. I was very skinny and tall while growing up. People would stop me on the street and ask if I had an eating disorder. (Why would anyone, and a perfect stranger at that, ask such a personal question?)

I soon discovered that being "me," which was skinny and tall, maybe wasn't the best thing. I even got it into my head that if I wasn't skinny that my assault would have never happened. Anyone who has been through trauma can understand that you go through the "woulda-shoulda-coulda's." I was never someone who cared how many calories were in a piece of chocolate cake. I grew up with parents who taught me to stop eating when I was full. So, I was always healthy no matter how skinny I was. My assault coupled with random people making rude comments to me affected the start of an eating disorder. Instead of starving myself, I started to overeat, and stuff myself with any food in sight. I was determined to be a larger sized girl. The flaw with my new found theory was I have always been active. I was in sports, I loved to dance and walk. I would walk everywhere. I was burning whatever I was eating. This was the beginning of bad food habits. These were new habits, ones that I didn't have as a kid.

I had to retrain my mind that it doesn't matter what people think about how I look. It matters what I think and how I feel. I had to ask myself, why I am I eating this whole bag of chips while watching Grey's Anatomy? Is it boredom? Am I sad? Am I hungry? Am I full? Usually my answer was, because I love barbecue chips! That answer was not good enough, even for this romantic. So, I had to ask again. That lead me to finish fast before I figured out the good answer, and had to put down the bag and pick up an apple! Self control was a constant battle. I still engage in this struggle every day. Sometimes I win, and sometimes I lose! Well, truthfully, I guess I always win in some way, shape, or form.

I am sure you have your own battle to fight. Perhaps it's not with food itself, but all it implies. This is when our wants and our needs collide. These two little guys don't always see eye-to-eye. My desire for a healthy body versus my need for a bag of chips conflicts quite often. In this first phase of the book, I will show you what to eat. This will, in turn, give you the benefits of losing weight (if you really need to,) better skin, shinier hair, longer nails, a sweet tasting little peach (your vagina) and great sex. Some simple foods combined with a little exercise will get you ready for the second phase, The Sexercises. Big Plus: it won't be a major downer, because let's be honest. The second you hear "diet" you automatically run for the hills. It's like a guy hearing the word "marriage!" We all have our individual fear of commitment, it just takes different forms.

What makes me qualified to tell you how to have a better sex life and body by what you eat? Well, I have sex, sometimes with a partner, but I also enjoy this activity with myself. Self love if you will. Mainly, what it comes down to is, I am a woman who really enjoys sexual activity. I am "in love" with being healthy, and want other women to share in this joy. My other qualification is I know what it feels like to not want to eat well, and to stuff your face with all the foods that you think will make you feel better. Eating this way is nice for the moment, but like any one night stand, in the morning you regret it!

Our bodies run on a different kind of love, but so do our individual exercise programs. Much like dating you have to find the right match. For sure, there's going to be the amazing first date and they don't call you ever again. You are left wondering, what did I do? Was it me? Why won't this work?

Then again, there is the person who you've been dating for months and still can't seem to get enough of them. They are perfect! Then, one night you wake up and anything can bother you about them. Like the very fact that they are breathing! As you kneel over him, staring at the drool rolling down his chin, clutching your pillow in both hands, you find yourself wondering whether it's time to silence their snoring, or break up.

It all comes down to the fact that there is a program out there for everyone, and not every program is for you. You should be happy with your choice. It should make you feel and look good. You shouldn't be embarrassed when you introduce your new lifestyle to your friends. They should be looking on in approval asking, "Does it have a brother/sister for me?"

My mother taught us kids a very simple and true rule: when you're full, stop eating. We heard none of the typical, "eat till your plate is clean." That's unhealthy. My siblings and I ate until we were full. We were also fortunate that we grew up in a happy household like this. Food was not about filling an unhappy void. I understand that happens a lot, and I have fallen prey to that in my adulthood. If you learn anything from this book, eat only until you are almost full, and enjoy the healthy food you are consuming.

I know from experience that when you're happy, you eat what is good for you and for your body. When you're unhappy, the opposite occurs. It's almost as if you subconsciously reinforce your unhappiness by making bad food choices. Let's work on getting you to a happier place, and a happier body!

Your Needs

"Serendipity. Look for something, find something else, and realize that what you've found is more suited to your needs than what you thought you were looking for."
- Lawrence Block

There are two things you will need to do:
Change Your Mindset
Find your Motivation

<u>Changing Your Mindset</u>

There comes a point in everyone's life when they say, "Tomorrow, I am going on a diet!" For some people this is a common occurrence. The issue is I am sure you will agree, diets do not work. I take that back. They work for a period of time, but after those few days, weeks or months they fall short of your overall goal. The only successful method is a lifestyle change. Food can be an addiction, plain and simple. You need it to survive. Sometimes it makes you "feel good" and sometimes it cheers you up. Your body is like the child and your mind is like the parent. You have to decide who is in charge, the child or the parent?

The first step is developing an effective mindset. You must love your body the way it is. Right now. Today. This mindset is something you will work on for the rest of your life. No two days in your life are the same. Today you may love your hips. Tomorrow, those hips could be your worst nightmare while wrestling your jeans to the floor after trying to fit them over your thighs. That's part of life. There is no simple way around it. I don't care how thin or heavy, or how tall or short you may be. Every woman, even super models and celebrities, feels bloated and unattractive at times.

I believe we all have something very much in common. We have all had, at one point or another, someone criticize us for how we look, or offer suggestions on how we can improve ourselves. I once had a boyfriend who wanted me to undergo breast augmentation. Obviously, he didn't love me or else he would not have asked me to do such a thing. I don't even have a small "rack" (which wouldn't be a bad thing,) but I'm not a Double D, either. In my opinion, I have an amazing set of lovely lady lumps. When I was living in California, I had people stopping me on the street to ask where I got my breasts "done." Only in Cali right? My reply was always, "God, my friends. God."

When it comes to our body we can become overly critical of ourselves, and of other people. We start to compare our body to someone else's in both positive and negative lights. "Oh, she is stick thin." "Wow, she really gained some weight since I saw her last." "I wish I had her nose."

We are all built differently, and that's what makes us each so beautiful. It's time to see what is beautiful in ourselves and in others. Own and embrace what you have, whatever that may be. Be happy for the person who has a figure like the one you desire. We would live in a better world if we would all love ourselves for whoever that person may be!

I don't believe in trying to change people or trying to mold someone to become the person you want. You love someone through thick and thin. Sure, there may be times when their habits may get on your very last nerve, but you have to choose your battles. (I'm going to go out on a very shaky limb and guess that you're not perfect, either. Who really is?) When it comes to changing ourselves, the only reason to do so is when it's for you, and only you. You are the person who has to live through, and with, any alterations. You have to be strong enough emotionally before any change to your body, mind or spirit can effectively take place. Wanting to grow as a person and human being is always commendable. A tip of the hat to you and your efforts! Just be sure it's for the right reasons.

Changing your mindset is hard to do in theory, but I think you'll find it easy with just a few pointers. Think about a time in the past when you believed in something strongly, and someone came along who said exactly the right thing to change your mind. Your mind was forever changed, wasn't it? What can you say to yourself that will forever change how you think? One way I have found to change my mindset is to decide that my body and I are in a romantic relationship. This isn't hard for my mind to believe in since, typically in the past, I was single and the only action I got was with myself! It's not that farfetched for me to convince my body that we are in a relationship. There are moments when it would seem we're in an abusive relationship, but I am always working on the balance! When you are in a loving, healthy relationship, don't you want that person to live forever? Aren't you planning on spending the rest of your life with them?

For example, one ex ate like he couldn't care any less whether he lived or died. When I started to believe we had some form of a future together, I started to freak out. I didn't want this guy to die on me, leaving me with five kids, a mortgage, and no sex! I immediately started incorporating salads and fresh fruit into his diet.

Ex-boyfriend's first reaction, "What's this green stuff? Ugh and why does it taste like grass?"

The answer was simple, "It's tastes like grass because it is grass. Kind of. I want to make sure we grow old together, which I'm afraid isn't going to happen if you continue eating the way you do."

Ex-boyfriend's reply, "If you keep feeding me stuff like this, there isn't going to be a future for us either."

That's where I learned that there is a delicate balance between eating healthy and treating yourself. The two must live in harmony, never feeling like the one is taking over the other. When it came down to it, my ex and I were opposites. I was healthy and he was like a treat.

This relationship didn't last because the treat didn't want the balance of being healthy. If you can learn to keep your romantic relationships healthy and in balance, you are on the right path for your body, too.

If you find your romantic relationships lacking in the healthy and balanced department, then may I suggest changing your mindset to believe that your body is a child. Would you feed a child a whole container of pre-made cookie dough? No, you would have a fun day making cookies and then after you ate your dinner, you would have some as a treat. When your "child" has been good, such as putting up with co-workers all week, or you've been to the gym three times this week, you may reward yourself with a fancy dinner and a glass of wine.

Change your mind set. Instead of thinking of how many calories are in the piece of chocolate cake, think about what would you give your child? Are you going to give your child that piece of cake? Possibly. Is it a special occasion like a birthday or wedding? Have you been eating so well that you just want to treat yourself? Are you too tired from work and you can't find the energy to make a proper dinner, and there is already a cake made up, just waiting on the table for a nibble? In my opinion, all reasons are valid. Sometimes it's a special occasion. Sometimes life is a celebration in itself, and sometimes it takes all your energy just to pick up the fork. I would like to believe you would feed your child in moderation. An example of a great rule my sister and her husband have come up with for their family is: Treats on Wednesdays and Saturdays. But, when any of the grandparents are around and want to give the kids treats, then it's ok. This rule is wonderful. It keeps you feeling like you get something for all your hard work, everything is still in good balance, and every now and then you'll feel spoiled.

Having a treat and being "spoiled" every now and then brings us to "cheating." What is it? Figure out how cheating is defined in your mind when it comes to your diet and don't do it, plain and simple. We all make sacrifices. When one gets married or is in a committed relationship, you make a promise to be true to your partner. You're committed to your body aren't you? The ground rules are set for what is considered cheating. Of course you're still going to enjoy life. Commitment is not a death sentence. You love the Opera and your partner doesn't? Not a bad thing, just go with a friend. You love fried chicken. Find a recipe that is still healthy but can satisfy your craving. If there are no healthy recipes out there for you, then now it's considered a treat. That means, have the fried chicken in moderation.

Find something that can satisfy your cravings without derailing you from your overall health goals. What can you live with, and what can't you live without? "Let your conscience be your guide," as my father would always say.

Motivation

What motivates you? What do you think will keep you motivated? To keep up with any health or exercise regimen, you need to have some form of motivation. It can be difficult to get to the gym. We are all busy and maybe even a little nervous. Sometimes it can be hard to keep the momentum going when we take breaks from our diet and fitness activities. Maybe we didn't do anything physical this past week or we skipped our spin/yoga/ stripper pole class. I've observed that many persons stop working out after a few days of "taking a break." Life becomes too busy and hectic and we say to ourselves, "I'll do it tomorrow." Next thing you know, a week has gone by, and we don't even know where our sneakers are hiding. Breaks are fine; just get yourself doing something after the time out. Even just one activity can get your mind back into taking care of your body.

Here are some motivators that I have been hearing from people lately.

I WANT TO:
Eat whatever I want
Wear whatever I want
Wear a strapless dress

I have a wedding or reunion coming up
It's bikini season
Vacation next month!

I want to set a good example for my children
I have health concerns
My body/heart/soul/psyche needs to heal

For me, one of my major motivators is love. I stay in shape for my significant other, and for the love of myself. It's a great motivator for my love not to want to take their eyes and hands off of me! If that means doing an extra Pilates session or even just 10 more minutes on the treadmill, I'm there. I also try to eat as healthily as possible for the love of my body, mind and soul. For me, sticking as close as I can to a clean diet, with no processed foods, is essential.

Now, when I'm not in a relationship, motivations become more short term and mainly support a pleasurable and satisfying life. Staying in shape so that I can eat as much as I want between Thanksgiving and New Years is a big one! Getting my butt to the gym because I'm going on vacation is another. Again, the focus is eating whatever I want. I'm a pleasure seeker. Good food, good wine and good love are my main focuses and motivations in life.

We all have moments when we feel unbelievably beautiful. Unfortunately, we also have moments when we feel disgusted with ourselves, and we vow to never again to finish a tub of ice cream in one sitting! Next time, we will take our time and finish it in two. It's a balancing act to stay healthy and happy. Sometimes the two do not mesh together easily, but certainly they should work together for the good of the body. For your ultimate success, your goals are to have a different mindset, and to have some form of motivation. In this phase, these are your only needs. Everything else will fall into place once you change your mindset and are motivated.

Dieting Around the World

"In spite of food fads, fitness programs, and health concerns, we must never lose sight of a beautifully conceived meal."
- Julia Child

Traveling, meeting new people and experiencing a new culture are passions of mine. I love waking up in a new city or town and not knowing all of the possibilities that await me outside my bedroom doors. I have yet to travel this whole world, so there is much for me yet to learn and to see. I have met many women (a few men) along my journey who I call my Mothers. They have taken me in when I needed a mother, since I was more than likely far away from my own little Mother. I have put together some of the diet tips they taught me in my travels. The one diet secret that was in common with all of my mothers from around the world: Life is to be enjoyed, and is too short for a diet!

Please remember this one diet secret, even if you don't remember anything else: Remember that life is to be enjoyed and is too short to not love life for all its splendors. Live like you only have this moment, but also take care of your body like you're going to live till 100.

French Mother: Drink Wine and Eat Good Fats.

It was early morning when I arrived in Brussels via a London train. This was my first time in Brussels. I was to stay with my cousin's friend, who became my French Mother. My eyes were sleepy but my heart was pounding with excitement. The city of Brussels was hustling and bustling. The sun was just coming up over this historic place. I arrived at my French Mother's townhouse and started to unpack. "This is all you have?" she asked me.

I try to travel light whenever I can. I also wanted to be able to bring a little something back to the States for my family and friends. Can't do a tour of Europe and not have at least a little gift for the ones you love! Every moment I got to spend with my French Mother was a delight. She was so smart and knowledgeable. I felt a connection with her instantly. Every night I would get home from my exploring and she would be cooking something so scrumptious I could hardly contain myself. Most of the meal's ingredients had been purchased just that day which is what you do in Europe. You always purchase fresh food every day. Every night during my visit with her we would talk about everything until very late in the evening. We would both realize what time it was and decide to get some sleep. In truth, I wanted to talk to her all night long. And when it came time for me to leave, I really didn't want to. I think of her always. Even though we only spent a few days together, she has had an enormous impact on my life. I will never be the same Dorothy again. For one of our meals she opened my eyes to Raclette, which is something the Swiss enjoy during their winter season. The set up is as follows: There is a special grill with multiple small pans that will be used to melt the slices of cheese. Once the cheese is melted and wonderfully gooey, pour over potatoes. My French Mother taught me an important lesson that day. "Never, ever, drink water when you are eating melted cheese. When the cheese and the water combined in your stomach you will end up with a terrible stomach ache because it is hard for the water to break down the cheese. Drink wine. The acidity in the wine helps to break down the cheese, which makes digestion easier." She didn't have to tell me twice to drink wine with dinner. I was all over it. "I drink a glass or two as often as I can. My husband knows more about wine than I do. I just love to drink it."

My French Mother also taught me to have a bit of good fat before each meal. A spoonful of olive oil or some nuts will do the trick.

Benefits of drinking wine

Reduces risk of death At least, most causes of mortality. Red wine has a protective effect on your body. Heart Disease It is well known that having a glass of red wine a day can keep the heart doctor away. Red wine reduces production of LDL (low density lipoprotein) and boosts HDL (high density lipoprotein) cholesterol.

Atherosclerosis: Not here! This is hardening of the arteries, usually caused when blood vessels are no longer able to relax. Red wine can help to relax blood vessels and help promote healthy blood flow.

Alzheimer's disease and Aging: There is a lower risk of Alzheimer's disease. Resveratrol is found in red wine, which can protect your brain and body against aging.

Heart Attacks: Having up to two glasses a day for women, and up to three a day if you're a man, can reduce your risk for a heart attack. Red wine can help a person to de-stress, which puts less strain on the heart.

Now, if you are someone who doesn't drink, you are still able to receive red wine's benefits. Here are a few ways: Eating red grapes on a regular basis. The skin of grapes contains many nutrients and antioxidants, just like the juice of the fruit. Peanuts also contain Resveratrol. These little nuts have a slightly higher amount of Resveratrol than grapes!

Remember, everything in moderation. This does not mean if you miss your glass of wine on Sunday, you can have three on Monday! Sorry, but it just doesn't work that way. If you are someone who is watching your weight, I suggest that instead of dessert you may have a glass of red wine.

If you don't already drink, there isn't a need to start. You may find yourself with a bad habit or gaining unwanted pounds since alcohol is "empty calories."

Benefits of good fats

Not only are good fats great for your hair, skin and nails, but good fats helps to stabilize cholesterol, improve the body's immune system and helps you to stay fuller longer. This aids in weight-loss, or at the very least, in stabilizing weight and overall health of the body. Even though good fats are good, remember that fats are still fats. So, everything in moderation. Just a few almonds before each meal will help you to lose weight and make you feel great!

Vietnamese Mother: Drink Tea and Eat Dark Chocolate

I woke up to the din of a crowd of voices. I thought, 'there must be a party going on downstairs!" I was staying with my one of my best friends, KitKat. I walked down the stairs to see what all the commotion was. I entered a small living room and about five of KitKat's little cousins where playing. Their mouths dropped open when they saw me. Standing at 5'10", I was by far the tallest person in the house at that moment. From the look on KitKat's cousins' faces, I may have been the first person of my height in this house, ever!

"Hello!" I gave a little wave. "Where is KitKat?" Their mouths still hadn't sprung back into place and they continued to stare at me. "Ok...well nice to see you. I'll go find her."

I walked into the kitchen where KitKat was watching her family play a card game. Everyone turned to me and gave me an up-and-down once over. I felt more awkward than usual and having just awakened, I wondered if my face had the imprint of the pillow and if my eyes had eye goo in them. Then, my Vietnamese Mother, KitKat's mother, ran right up to me and gave me a big hug. "How was your nap? Are you hungry? I'll make you something. Here, have some tea first. Prepares the body to eat."

As I sipped on my tea, I was introduced to the whole family. Well, the small portion of the family who was at the house that day. I heard an aunt say something in Vietnamese. KitKat turned to me and said, "She said you look like Jessica Simpson." I quickly smiled, since I think Jessica is beautiful, "Thank you!"

Whenever I visit KitKat her family is so welcoming and warm. Her mother and father always offer me something to eat when I enter their home. It makes me feel like I'm back with my family. Sometimes, KitKat will protest in Vietnamese, while her Mother is trying to feed me one of her special dishes, "No, Mother, we are leaving soon. We're going to eat out tonight." I just smile and nod but part of me wants to stay in and eat her mother's cooking. It's beyond tasty and healthy. Plus, how can I say no to the special shrimp dish she makes?

While watching a movie with KitKat, my Vietnamese Mother will come in to check on us and see if there is anything that we need. "Would you like some soup? I will pour you some tea." She will leave the room and come back with tea for the both of us and a bowl of chocolates to share. "It's dark chocolate. I eat this every day, keeps me young and healthy and it makes me smile." Her Mother says, overjoyed.

KitKat's mother is maybe the sweetest woman on the planet, and probably the cutest. Aside from her disposition, she is a very smart little mother and keeps her family eating well. Through her cooking she has a very healthy, satisfied, and happy family indeed.

Benefits of drinking tea
Drinking tea before you begin to consume food will help prepare the body for digestion. Tea also may aid in the body's elimination of waste and toxins. Tea also contains anti-oxidants, boosts immune system in the blood, and boosts metabolism. Drinking five cups a day of

green tea can help one to burn up to 80 additional calories.

Benefits of eating dark chocolate daily

There are benefits to eating dark chocolate. I suggest around three ounces a day. Not only do you get your chocolate fix, and I'm sure that will put a smile on your face, but chocolate may help you to lose weight. Eating something sweet like fruit or chocolate sends a signal to the brain that you are full and the meal is complete. Dark chocolate increases endorphin production. When a female eats chocolate it stimulates the same pleasure section in the brain as sex does. Chocolate may also be an anti-depressant since it contains serotonin. Also, dark chocolate has a small amount of caffeine, which helps to ease PMS issues.

Italian Mother: Olive Oil

"I have olive oil with every meal. Everyone in my family loves olive oil. It's a staple. We dip bread in it, we cook with it and we even drink it. Olive oil is life." My Italian Mother is everything you would want in an "Italian Mother." She is warm, a great cook and has great fashion sense. I've noticed that Europeans have a way of speaking and conversing that makes life that much more beautiful. They really do know how to enjoy life, at least it would seem this way. Their priorities are different than those of Americans. Americans want wealth and fame and we want it yesterday. Everything is so fast for us. I found in Italy, life is fast, but in a different way. It's a land where eating habits become social, family is number one, and driving slowly is not optional!

One of my favorite moments with my Italian Mother was when we went shopping. Actually, we weren't supposed to be shopping. We were supposed to be meeting up with the family and we were late. "Ok, Hun, we have less than ten minutes. Stick with me, I'll show you how it's done." We continued into the store and my Italian

Mother moved with fury. Never have I seen anyone move that fast and still be that graceful. She was like a lioness hunting her prey. She picked out a few items she liked and moved right to the check-out. We were in and out in less than ten minutes. I was impressed and vowed I would learn all that I could from this woman.

She taught me hints about many things: How to make a yummy, gooey lasagna, how to choose the right man ("He has to love you more than anything my dear!") and about olive oil. "Olive oil is life," as my Italian Mother has said. She typically will have a spoonful in the morning, a spoonful when she's hungry but can't eat yet, and a spoonful before bed.

Benefits of Olive Oil

Olive oil is great for the skin, hair and nails. It has been known for centuries that this oil can slow the aging process and help with arthritis. This oil also contains other health benefits. If you have a spoonful of olive oil when you wake up, and have another spoonful before bed, it will help aid the body's elimination process of waste and toxins. If you are ever feeling hungry, this oil will actually help you to curb your hunger and cravings. So, when you are reaching for pint of ice cream, maybe fill your spoon up first with some olive oil. Wait a minute for your brain to realize its full, and hopefully you won't overdo it on the Chunky Monkey. All of these benefits are key to a healthy, fit body.

Mexican Mother: Love and Avocados

"I tell those I love that I love them. Americans hold back the telling of love, when they shouldn't." One of my boyfriends, who grew up in Mexico, and I were together for only one week before he told me he loved me, and I told him I loved him. It was normal. In America, if you tell someone that you love them they run away, even though they may love you back. Makes no sense. No wonder Americans have more cases of illness. You hold everything in. You don't share the happy moments and you stew in the sad moments. "Things happen, Dorotee. Life happens. All we have is love." This is what my Mexican Mother said to me on one of our first encounters. I knew then, we were always going to be in each other's lives. She is younger than I am, but age doesn't matter when it comes to the heart. She is always there for me, protecting me, and if needs be, fighting for me. That sounds like a mother to me. Her key to staying healthy is eating good-for-you food like avocados, putting love into all of her cooking, and saying "I love you" to who she loves every day, as many times a day as she can.

Benefits of Avocados

Avocados contain the good fats that we love for healthy hair, skin and nails. Healthy fats also help one to lose weight. Avocados also contain vitamin E which is essential to the body's health. Avocados have been known to help prevent cancer, especially prostate, breast and oral cancers. So, maybe it's time to have an avocado a day. I don't know about you, but I love fresh guacamole.

Benefits of saying "I love you"

Saying I love you to someone actually helps to form a bond between the two persons. Endorphins are released in both persons' brains when you say or hear "I love you." Saying I love you is both beneficial to the person saying this phrase, but also beneficial to the person receiving it. This simple phrase may boost your immune system as well as boost your metabolism. These benefits aid in weight-loss as well as over-all body function and health. So, start telling those you love that you love them...everyday...all day!

Portuguese Mother: Eat Little Meals, Be Social and Take Your Time

"When I eat it's because I need to eat. I need the food that I am about to put in my body. When I go out to eat, it's an experience. I'm there to be with friends and family. If I'm by myself, I'm there to be with myself and enjoy my own company. I take my time. There is no rush to get back to work because the work will still be there when I get back to my office. You Americans, everything is so fast, so quick. You are all in such a rush to eat. You don't actually experience what you are eating. What is the point of eating, if you're just going to gobble up your meal? No, I take my time and enjoy my meal. Enjoy time with my family and friends. What is the point to life anyway? Are we put on this earth to slave away all day at a desk? I hope not."

I met my Portuguese Mother while visiting Oporto, Portugal. It is a city that still closes down on Sundays and most businesses are small, family-owned-and-run. She helped me out quite a bit while I was visiting her city: She told me what sites to see, where to eat, and how to make a group of dogs stop following me around the city. This last tip was extra helpful since I was a few moments away from adopting each puppy and   bringing them back to the states with me!

There was one restaurant in particular that she shared with me. It was around the corner from where I was staying. As I was deciding on what I was going to have for dinner, she told me how her family eats. "Only eat a little bit at a time. You take one bite and put down your fork or spoon. Chew your food, listen to the conversation, have a sip of wine. Then you may take another bite and start the process all over again. Don't rush your meal and pay attention to what is going on around you. If you don't you could miss something." She also told me that taking a nap everyday was the key to good health. "It's not just for babies. Everyone needs a nap."

Benefits of eating slowly

When one eats slowly it allows more time for the brain to send the "full" signal to the stomach to stop eating. This allows your body to only consume what it needs in the way of substance. So, eat slowly. You will eat fewer calories which will aid in weight-loss, or will result in no weight gain. Also, one will take the time to enjoy the food that is placed before them. Enjoy your food, enjoy your life.

Benefits of Taking a Nap

There are so many health benefits to taking a cat nap that I am really surprised that it's not part of our everyday life. In fact, I sense that it's frowned upon in the states to take a nap. The belief seems to be that you are lazy for taking a nap. The benefits, in my opinion, outweigh the dirty looks you will receive. Taking a cat nap reduces stress, and aids in heart health. A nap allows you the time to stay focused at work and boosts creativity. Napping also burns calories and allows the body to have a higher rate of cell turnover. So, if you want a slimmer waistline, less stress in your life, and better skin? Take a cat nap.

Brazilian Mother: Pineapple

I met my Brazilian Mother while shopping one day. Actually, my Brazilian Mother isn't a woman, but a gay man. He isn't offended when I call him my Brazilian Mother. On the contrary, he likes it when I call him Hot Momma. He helped me pick out a pair of shoes and a dress for a party that I was attending. During the minutes between finding out my shoe size (size 7) and finding out my dress size (size 6) we became friends. Not sure how I reeled this little 5'5" Brazilian hottie in, but I am so happy that I did. Not only has he helped me fashion-wise, but he has opened my eyes to many diet secrets that have helped me to stay slim. At the top of the list? Eating pineapple after a meal. "Giselle does this, baby. Everyone in Brazil does this, baby." I have no idea if Giselle eats pineapple. She could be allergic to pineapple for all I know. His Brazilian accent is very thick, which for some reason makes me believe that Giselle does eat pineapple after every meal! How else could she stay so thin after eating a hamburger and fries for lunch?

Benefits of Eating Pineapple

Pineapples contain Bromelain which is an enzyme that aids digestion. One may take a Bromelain tablet instead of fresh pineapple, and this should be taken in between meals to aid digression. Pineapple also contains vitamin C which boosts immune system function and helps with anti-aging. My suggestion is to eat pineapple in between meals as a healthy snack. Do not eat with other foods in order to receive the full benefits.

Irish Mother: Bananas and Laugh All Day

I had met my Irish Mother while I was playing with a child I was babysitting. We hit it off right away. She has such a great laugh and smile, they're infectious. One day while we were catching up at her house, she told me about her large family back in Ireland. "All we do is laugh! Oh we love beer, but who doesn't love beer?" She said this to me in a slight Irish brogue. Being in the states for as long as she has been, she's lost most of her accent. The only time I would hear it come out in full force was when I went with her to Ireland and spent some time with her beautiful family. While catching up with my Irish Mother, she said she was going to make herself a smoothie, did I want one as well? I never pass on a smoothie, so I said yes please! She started to prepare the smoothie and turned to me, "You know I started putting a banana in my smoothies. I've noticed that when I do, I feel fuller longer. It could just be in my head, but I have noticed a change in my hunger and how I act throughout the day. I don't eat as much. Do you want a banana in your smoothie?" I thought about it for a moment and decided to try my own experiment. "Yes please. Thank you for the smoothie!"

We enjoyed our smoothie and laughed the afternoon away until it was time for me to head home for dinner. My first thought when I arrived at my house was, "Oh my goodness, I'm not hungry and I have plenty of energy. I may even go for a run." Then I remembered I don't like to run, so I went for a walk on the beach instead.

Benefits of Laughing

Laughing speeds your heart rate, releases muscle tension, and increases the amount of oxygen in your blood. It also produces the happy drug in the brain called endorphins. In theory, if you laughed for 15 minutes every day, you'd burn enough calories to lose one pound a year. Laughing burns 1.5 calories per minute. So the more you laugh, the more weight you will lose. That is amazing!

Benefits of Bananas

Not only does a banana help in making a smoothie thicker and creamer, but it also contains health benefits. The biggest benefit that most people already know is that bananas contain potassium. Potassium aids in the body's overall health, especially with heart function. Bananas also help to stabilize your mood. Bananas contain the highest amount of B6, which helps to stablize blood sugars. Bananas contain fiber. Add bananas to your breakfast, combined with a nutbutter for a midday snack, or add it to your fruit smoothie.

My French Great-Grandmother: Eat Fresh, Clean Foods

I wasn't named after Dorothy from Oz. I was named after my great-grandmother, Dorothy, or "Ma" as the rest of my family and I refers to her. She is a little French woman standing at 4'9" with hair and heels. Just the cutest thing you have ever seen. I remember walking into her house when I was younger and seeing her vacuum in stiletto heels. I thought to myself, "I want to be like that!" For years now, when anyone would speak to my Ma she would just smile, nod and say "Yes". She has had trouble hearing for quite some time now. She's didn't want to be

disagreeable. It wouldn't matter what you were saying to her, she would just smile and nod so very sweetly.
My Ma's backyard was full of flowers and shade trees, but the majority of the backyard was a large fruit and vegetable garden. The freshest, tastiest fruits and vegetables came from my Ma's garden.   Ma was quite the gardener. To this day, her homemade pickles can't be beat and her tomatoes are the juiciest. Nothing compares to her homemade strawberry jam. In her younger years, if she didn't grow it, then she didn't eat it. She grew up during the Great Depression, when food and money were scarce. She learned at a young age to grow and can her own fruits and vegetables. Some say because she didn't grow up with processed foods, this was the reason for her living so long. She was healthy and was able to stay independent until just a few months before she passed away at the age of 99.

Benefits of eating fresh fruits and vegetables
   Fresh fruits and veggies are a must for weight-loss and overall body health. Not only do fresh fruits and veggies contain fiber, but some actually contain protein, such as peas. Start your own little garden today. Nothing tastes as good as your own fresh tomato sauce. Plus, the money saved from having your own garden will allow you to take a trip, or to treat yourself to a manicure!
   Gardening is also a great stress reliever for some people. It allows you time in the sun (Vitamin D) and a way to be with nature. It also is a great way to feel like you have accomplished something. While I lived in San Diego, I had a mini garden on my balcony. I grew herbs and some veggies. I was so proud of myself when my first cucumber showed up. Honestly, it felt like I could accomplish anything after that. Funny, how growing your own food will do that to your ego.

Benefits of Clean Foods (Not processed)

The benefits of having a clean diet not only extend to weight-loss, but also to your hair, skin and nails. The chemicals in processed foods may dull skin and hair. Once you cut out anything processed, your body's weight will stabilize, you will have more energy, and you may even find you have a happier disposition and attitude.

Benefits of Making Your Own Junk Food

I do not know many people who are able to stay completely away from junk food. So, what about making your own? They will not have as many chemicals and won't be as processed as store-bought. Start making your own potato chips, cookies and ice cream. You may find a new outlet for stress (I find when I bake, I am at peace with myself.) You will be helping to keep you and your loved ones healthy, as well as satisfied.

My Own Mother: Dessert

Growing up we didn't eat a lot of junk. Every now and again my parents would order a pizza and we were allowed to have a glass of soda. We didn't eat or drink this type of food on a regular basis. I don't even remember going to any fast food places as a child, only when we asked for our birthday parties to be at any particular fast food chain. It wasn't normal to eat junk. When I wanted a snack my Mother would say, "Have a piece of fruit or a piece of cheese." My Mother cooked well-balanced meals for all of us (six) children and my 6'6" tall father. She did, however, have dessert treats for us! These treats were always homemade. It was way too expensive for her to do it any other way when I was a child. For six little scavengers you had to watch the food budget. A phrase I recall hearing from my father was, "If it's healthy, then kids probably don't want to eat it. So, find out what the kids hate and give them plenty of it." My Mother's only rule when it came to us eating treats was, "If you have a little bit of dinner, then you may have a little bit of dessert." I often remember asking what we were having for dinner, and if I wasn't happy with the answer, quickly following up with, "What are we having for dessert?" Sometimes this rang true with what my Mother cooked. Healthy, well balanced meals. So, if I knew we were going to have a tasty dessert then I could handle dinner.

Five Year Old Self: "I'm full."
Parents: "Just a few more bites."
Five Year Old Self: "Ok, may I have dessert?"
Father: "You said you were full."
Five Year Old Self: "Well, I'm full from dinner, but I left this much room for dessert." (I put my hands into a small circle and placed it on my belly.)

Benefits of Balancing Dinner and Dessert
  I don't know about you, but there are times when I am not in the mood for a regular dinner, I want a piece of chocolate cake. Knowing that I am in the mood for dessert, I try to keep that in mind when I am planning my dinner. I plan on eating enough to get the nutrients that I need for a healthy body and then leave room for dessert. This is a delicate balance since how do you know how much room will be needed for that yummy piece of chocolate cake? Eat slowly and have time between dinner and dessert. This allows your brain plenty of time to determine how much dessert that the body will be able to handle without stuffing your body and making you have that icky feeling of over-eating. My Mother's rule of thumb, if you have a little bit of dinner than you may have a little bit of dessert. So if you only have half a salad and a piece of chicken. For dessert you may have 3oz of dark chocolate. Per what my Father would always say to my siblings and me, "Let your conscience be your guide." It's a nice rule of thumb for sure.

Scandinavia Mother: Eat Whatever, and Enjoy Talking About Sex, and Having Sex

  "Sex is so taboo in America. You Americans are how do you say...Prudes? It's not a big deal to talk about sex, to walk around naked, or to have sex. It's natural. From a young age, we are taught our bodies are natural and beautiful. If a man sees your breasts at the beach, it's not a big deal. He doesn't stare and make you feel uncomfortable." My response was, "Well, maybe it's good that we Americans are more prudish. Whenever my old boyfriend would see my breasts, his eyes would bulge right out of his head and he would say it felt like Christmas. Can't beat that compliment!"

My Scandinavia Mother has a rock solid body, is over 40, and a blonde, blue eyed beauty. She doesn't "work out" and she doesn't "diet." What does she do to stay to healthy? "I live life and I eat well. I don't deny myself something I want. If I want pasta, I eat pasta. I don't work out, but I go swimming or find some other activity I enjoy." Maybe it's her good genes, but I have a sneaky suspicion that it's her outlook and her energy that keeps her looking so amazing.

Benefits of Sex
Sex is by far my favorite subject. I love to talk about it. For me, it is completely normal to discuss sex, since it is one of my passions and obsessions. Sex is healthy. Sex is natural. The benefits of sex are so long I could write a whole book on just sex alone. (Maybe I will.) Not only does sex provide great exercise for toning your muscles and burning calories, but on average, sex burns about 300 calories in an hour. This includes kissing, foreplay and intercourse, oh my. Intercourse is a great way to stretch and tone your whole body, sometimes muscles you didn't even realize that you had. If you're feeling guilty about eating that piece of cake or that pound of bacon, maybe it's time to grab your honey and do the "No Pants Dance". Or just dance by yourself. That burns calories and tones your body as well. You don't need a partner to get the benefits of sex.

Benefits of Eating What You Want

Amazing Love Diet

For me, when I've been on diets in the past and I'm not allowed to eat a certain food or have a particular drink, that food or beverage becomes all I can think about. When one limits oneself, you destroy free will and your freedom to do what brings you joy in this world. While it is true everything should be in moderation, knowing that it makes you gain weight also may help not feeling sad about not being able to eat a certain food. Think of it as being allergic to the food that causes you to gain weight. Listen to your body. I know that I love beer, but it makes me feel sick, and causes my stomach to blow up like a balloon. I try to stay away from beer as much as possible, even though sometimes that's all I want to drink on a hot summer day. Eat what you want, but know that there are limits when it comes to your body and your overall health.

Eat, Drink & Be Merry

"Nothing would be more tiresome than eating and drinking if God had not made them a pleasure as well as a necessity."

-Voltaire

Amazing Love Diet

There was a moment in my life when I realized that, sometimes, food is better than sex, or at the very least, it's comparable. I was having dinner with my one of my best friends. My closest friends and I share many of the same interests. We enjoy the great pleasures in life. The consumption of good food and great wine is something we enjoy together. I don't really remember what myself and this particular friend had to eat that night, but it was incredible. I'm sure we started with one or two amazing appetizers followed up with a tantalizing fish entrée, and an amazing bottle of red wine. My friend is very good at choosing wine. She learned by traveling and tasting wines all over the world.

We finished our meals with a smoldering, chocolate lava cake oozing with chocolaty goodness. After the last bite, we both sat back quite sated, and looked at each other, not saying a word. It was one of the best meals either of us had ever had and words could not describe the joy our bodies were feeling. It wasn't just a meal but was a completely satisfying experience in so many ways, at least for me. I can't speak for my friend, but judging from the look on her face, she felt the same way as I did. For another several minutes, I don't think we moved. We couldn't. Our bodies had released so many happy endorphins and euphoric feelings that our minds had to shut down in order to take it all in. Honestly, I don't know if I could handle having a meal like that every day. My body would go into stimulated overload because of the pure joy my taste buds would be feeling.

It was comparable to some of my best orgasms. You know the kind, or if you don't you soon will, where after you can't move, think or speak. Sometimes you have enough energy to listen or feel your own heartbeat beating quickly in your chest, and you take in a deep breath to try to collect yourself. But, that's all that your mind can handle at that moment in time. This feeling was that meal. Couldn't move, couldn't speak, and certainly I was completely satisfied. It was most definitely a multiple-orgasmic meal, if you will.

This got me to thinking. If food could cause multiple orgasms of the taste buds in our mouths, then perhaps this could be a major reason why some women who are so unsatisfied sexually turn to food. Heck, I would, and sometimes do! There are two men in this world who have never let me down, and who can always satisfy a craving or two: Ben and Jerry. Curling up with them and a romantic movie is a great night to me. That is, of course, until I start not fitting into my jeans. That's when that relationship goes sour. We start to fight. I say, never again will I be fooled by you, never again. Really? Food can be a love/hate relationship, but it doesn't have to be. You can have your cake and eat it too! Just not all at once, and not all the time

When I think "diet," I think of a quick fix. When I hear "lifestyle change," I hear big commitment and torture. From my observation, most people have similar beliefs. Isn't there a healthy routine that doesn't require me giving up everything I love, all for the sake of a conventional "perfect" body? I was overjoyed for my body, my soul and my mind when I found it. I could love my body inside and out, and reach the goals I was so desperately trying to obtain with greater success than I had had in the past.

Treating your body with love is the key to a healthy body. Example: If you are pregnant, and are committed with love to have a healthy baby, you will do all the things you're supposed to do when you're pregnant to ensure that end. You eat non-processed foods, lots of fruit and veggies, lean proteins, and take your daily vitamins. If you take that approach with your body, thinking of this as a "gestational" project, you'll find your body is "developing" into shape and you look and feel great.

Amazing Love Diet

What would you feed your child? Most parents want their children to eat what is best for them, but the parent herself may tend to skip meals, eat unhealthy foods, and or to eat on the run. Do you want your children to develop unhealthy eating habits? I would hope not. The best way to ensure that your child eats healthily is to monitor what they consume. My suggestion is to do the same for you. When growing up, it was only on special occasions like birthdays or holidays that we were allowed to consume unhealthy portions of foods. We always had dessert. If we just ate a little dinner, then we got a little dessert. It was balanced. (The exceptions were anytime a grandparent gave us ice cream for breakfast, and the night we decorated our Christmas tree!)

When it comes to breaking a habit, all we are really doing is starting up another (hopefully healthy) habit to take its place. An example: substitute dark chocolate for milk chocolate. It's higher in antioxidants.

There is no right time to start a diet, but there are always plenty of excuses not to: "If I start now, I'll miss all the holiday parties." Or, my favorite, "After this weekend, I'll start my diet." You will always fail with this attitude. Just start now. Doesn't mean you give up on carbs and wine altogether. Just consume these treats in moderation. Are you heading to a big party this Saturday? Perfect! Have a game plan before you put on your party dress. That's why I take my eating experiences as they come, one day at a time. Just because you're not on a conventional diet doesn't mean you shouldn't eat well today, or that it gives you a free pass to eat whatever you want, anytime you want. You are alive aren't you? Time to act like it! What you put in your mouth should be for a very good reason. There is a way to balance eating healthy and eating happy.

I have mentioned before about motivation and love. When it comes to most of what I eat I eat certain foods knowing they are going to help my love life. Everything is connected. And I mean this in every sense of the word. If you eat a piece of fruit, it nourishes your body. It makes its way through your system and provides your body with the benefits of vitamins, pectin for your arteries' health, and wonderful fiber. But, this piece of fruit helps in other ways as well. I am sure you've heard of aphrodisiacs, right? Certain foods help to turn you on and get you in the mood for sex. Well, this is true! But, did you also know there are foods that can make sex better for you and your partner, as well as make you look more attractive?

Here is a list of foods that help your body as a sexual being:

Fats

Olive oil, Grapeseed Oil, Avocado oil, Avocados, Chia seeds and flax seed. These are great, and rich in the types of healthy fats you want for your skin and hair. They help to get the blood flowing to the right areas, if you know what I mean.

Fruits
Any fruit is good for your body, but these are the best:
Fruit sweetens you literally. You will have a sweeter taste and smell in your nether region.
Apples - Great benefits
Strawberries
Oranges - Great benefits
Grapes
Apricots
Bananas
Peaches

Veggies and Legumes
These are the best! Bright colors, as well as green, are best for your sexual body.

Avocado
Carrots - Helps to give you a great glow and it is a natural at fighting harmful rays from the sun.
Celery - Great for your bones. It is said that the resulting smell your skin will secrete makes you more attractive sexually.
Cucumbers
Eggplant
Tomato
Beans
Garlic
Leeks
Onions
Peppers
Soybeans
Spinach
Sweet potatoes
Lentils
Beets
Winter squash

Protein

Some vegetables and grains contain protein. The best sources of protein, in my opinion, are fish, beans, eggs, lean chicken or turkey. If you love meat like steak and burgers, keep these to twice a month, maybe when you are feeling yourself getting weak, or if you just love meat and need to meet a craving. Too much red meat causes the taste of your genitals and skin to be bitter and sour.

Salmon is the best
Sardines, if you can stand them
Seafood, Shrimp, Scallops, Oysters (Oysters have a special power. It is not true what they say about them being an aphrodisiac, but they will help you to climax faster)
Eggs, egg yolks are great for you.
Eel (If you like sushi)
Kidney beans

Black beans
Soy
Tofu
Seeds: Pine nuts and pumpkin
Nuts like cashews, almonds and walnuts

Grains
Your grains are not limited to just the following. I love quinoa and I think it is such a power food.
Quinoa
Brown Rice
Steal Cut Oats

What to drink
Lots of water to flush out your system, and to keep your skin hydrated and glowing
Teas such as green, white or nettle (Nettle tea has certain qualities that aid the vagina's scent)
Alcohol dulls the skin, but having a glass of red wine has many benefits and those benefits increase during the hours of happy hour, believe it or not.   Having a glass between the hours of 4-8 is a good thing. (But, why limit "Happy" to just an hour?)

Miscellaneous

Benefits of Chia Seeds:

-Makes you feel fuller longer: So if you don't want to add calories but you want to feel full and have health benefits this is your magic food.
-Balance Blood Sugar: Slows down the body's conversion of starches into sugars.
-Omega-3s and 6: By weight, Chia seeds contains more omega 3 than salmon and flax seeds.
-Protein: 1 tablespoon of Chia seeds contains 2 grams of protein. Chia seeds are a complete protein, so no need to combine with other foods.
-Fiber: 1 tablespoon contains 5.5 grams of fiber

-Fight Aging: Chia seeds are packed with anti-oxidants.
-Vitamins: Contains calcium, magnesium, copper, iron, zinc and many more!
-Easy to Digest: Unlike flax seeds these beauties don't need to be ground up. Can sprinkle on everything if you really wanted to.
-Energy: The health pioneer Paul Bragg did an experiment an endurance hike with friends. They divided up into a Chia-eating group and another group, who ate whatever they wanted. The group eating only Chia seeds finished the hike four hours, twenty-seven minutes before the others, most of whom didn't even finish at all.
-Substitute: Use the Chia gel for baking!
-Clean: It helps to cleanse the intestines.
-Weight-loss: The combination of feeling fuller and cleansing the body equals a slimmer waistline.
So this magic food helps to keep your body in tip top condition, keeps you looking young, vibrant and feeling your best!

Dark chocolate is the best and has antioxidants, which I have discussed before. Enjoying 3 oz with a few almonds mixed in is great. This amount of chocolate is just the right amount. Dark chocolate has many known benefits, but it also can help put your body in the mood, and help you lose weight. If you can't do straight-up dark, do Chuaho chocolate pods. They are 60% dark. You may find more information on their website, www.chuaochocolatier.com.

Salty and fried foods can make skin and hair look dull and it can make it difficult to achieve orgasm. (They can affect you so negatively that you do not have an orgasm. No joke!!! So try to stay away from salty and fried food. You want your plate to be colorful with as many colors as the rainbow. (Talk about eating happy!)

Here is an example of what I think your plate should look like:

(I drew this example...I'm not an artist, as you can tell.)

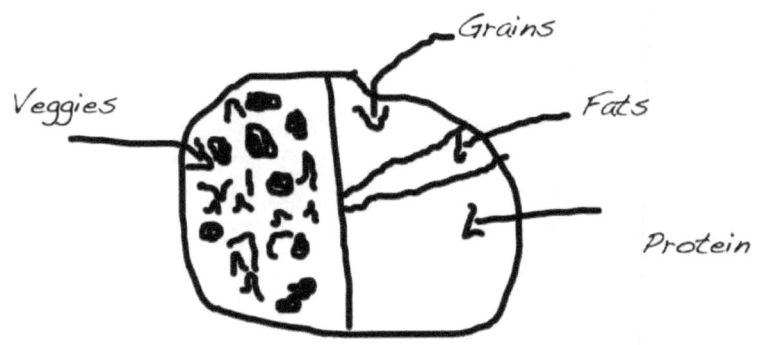

Some foods that may be harmful to your sexual body
    In particular, dairy. This is just my opinion, but here is some of the research that I found. Don't go by what I say, though, make your own educated decision. Some people very close to me will never give up dairy. Every now and again, I cook with it. How else am I to make delicious whipped cream? The following are not meant to scare you, or deter you from eating dairy. I have included them to make you think about what you put in your body just because someone else told you it was healthy.

-After the age of three the human body stops being able to break down dairy products.

-The African Bantu consume about 350mg of calcium per day. They rarely have a broken bone or lose their teeth and there is no calcium deficiency.

-Americans consume about 1000mg of calcium per day

-Native Eskimos consume about 2000mg of calcium per day and have the highest rate for Osteoporosis in the world!

Here are some of my favorite alternatives to dairy
-Soy Milk, Soy Cheese, Soy Yogurt, Soy Ice Cream (Soy may lower men's libidos. I have also found that I tend to gain a pound or two eating soy. Everyone is different. Test and   experience for yourself.)
-Rice Milk, Rice Cheese (not as "plastic" as it used to be!)
-Almond Milk (Huge fan!)
-Hemp Milk, Hemp Cheese

        If you follow this diet you will have no problem finding balance within your body. These foods help to naturally shed weight, will benefit your sex life, and make you glow with health and happiness. If you stick to fewer processed foods, eat fresh fruits and veggies, you will find your body improves, and your sex life will, too. Everything within your body is connected. If you are missing one part of the puzzle, it cannot be complete. Eating right is a special puzzle piece that people often forget about and neglect. Start today by putting the right foods in your body. When your body is in balance everything else finds its balance, as well. Within no time you'll be feeling better about yourself, and enjoying life to the fullest.

"In my end is my beginning."

-T.S. Eliot

When I truly listen to my body and supply its needs, I find myself easily being happy, fit and feeling good about how I look. The human mind is the best machine ever invented. Sure, there are a few glitches here and there. From time to time, faulty software has been downloaded. Just download a software upgrade and you'll be back in business. When I listen to my body, I know I will have an upset stomach when I drink milk. My body becomes bloated when I eat tofu, and my knees hate lunges. What should I do? I should adapt. It's survival. I try to avoid milk and tofu. When I work out I find an exercise that targets those muscle groups that my body will be able to handle in substitute for the lunges. So, listen to your body. Sometimes what you need to change is as simple as one thing. Other times it's a complete life, or physical, overhaul.

Having a healthy, fit body means more than a healthy diet and exercise. The largest component to a healthy body is the one that most people tend to forget about, or disregard, the mind. If you don't have a healthy mind and spirit you're doing your overall body's health a disservice. You'll over- or under-work your body and mind if these two aspects of your Self are not in balance.

I don't like the idea of depriving myself. I understand religious reasoning, (i.e.: Giving something up for your spiritual well-being.) Fasting can clear your mind of "wants," or at the very least, help you to feel closer to God. Most of us earthlings too often deprive ourselves of something, then turn around and act out in destructive ways. What is happiness? What is beautiful? The two are, more often than not, connected.

Outer beauty is fleeting and takes place in a finite period of time. Real beauty is within and lasting. Why do we want to be beautiful? The answer (that I have come up with) boils down to finding a suitable mate. My theory is, it is our human instinct to find a mate and reproduce. Nowadays, what is really beautiful has been skewed by the media and Hollywood. These two powerful forces have embedded little ticking time bombs into our brains. They make us believe that to be beautiful means to be thin, have large breasts, perfect skin, no rolls of fat, wrinkles, or visible cellulite, and do this all while wearing the latest fashion! The end result is, if you follow the mainstream beliefs, everyone will end up looking and being exactly the same. We would resemble little cookie-cutter people walking down the street, single file.

When I was young and fretting about an outfit, or worried about what others might think of me, my mother used to say, "What's the worst thing that could happen? They might laugh at you? Then you made someone happy. If you can live with the worst thing that could happen, go for it! It doesn't matter what other people think."

Our current society doesn't like change and it certainly doesn't embrace the term "different." Imagine a world where you could be truly yourself and accepted for it. Today, to receive this sort of acceptance, someone has to be in love with you. I long for the day when people will feel free to wear what makes them feel good and not to care if lines are starting to show up on their faces. I have observed that the older someone is the more they tend to come into their own. They no longer want to keep up with the Joneses, and are more secure with the way they look. Every day is a struggle for me. Some days I feel wonderful, beautiful and witty! Within 24 hours, I could discover none of my clothes fit me, I want to hide my face, and somehow, when I open my mouth all that seems to come out is gibberish and nonsense!

It is my belief that when we enter this world, we have a job to do, or a life purpose, which can bring us (and others) great joy. It is also my belief that we know or have an idea of what our life purpose is when we our young. If you look back to your childhood, what were your interests, your talents? Try to remember, what was the main thing that brought joy to your life? Speaking for myself, I had many interests. I loved to write plays and music, sing, dance and I was always trying to invent something new. Even with all of these interests, there was one topic that stood out to me, Love.

It wasn't really an interest as much as it was a calling in Life. I knew deep down in my soul that I wanted it, even though I didn't really know what it was, or what it entailed. We are all born with a certain, God-given purpose, and there are certain things that we need to achieve within our lifetime. Maybe you were born to be the mother of an activist, or maybe you were born to travel the world. Everyone's purpose is just as important as the next person's. Being the President of the United States is just as important as being a housewife in Omaha, Nebraska. Why? Because everything we do in this world within our own lifetime has an effect on the future, and on someone else. So, to say one person is more important than another is just not the truth. Sometimes, even the way we die is our purpose in life. Tragic accidents happen all the time. Sometimes, even though a tragedy did happen, it results in changes to laws, there will be more safety precautions taken, and lives will be ultimately being saved.

Figure out what brings you joy in this world. We are merely a flicker of light, and our life here is precious and no monetary value may be placed on it. Time is short, but always high in demand. We always want more of it, and we always think we have another day.

Grateful

"Promise me you'll always remember: You're braver than you believe, and stronger than you seem, and smarter than you think."

-Christopher Robin to Pooh, A.A. Milne

I am so very grateful that I was able to write this book. It has been a dream of mine for years and now it's a reality. I have been lucky enough to have the love and support of my family and friends. In return, I am very lucky to have a family I love and cherish. They are my world. I am also very fortunate to have friends who I would do almost anything for, and who would do the same for me. Never in my life have I felt as loved as I do at this very moment. I am surrounded by love. Because I am loved and supported, I am able to do anything, especially in my efforts to keep my body healthy.

Sometimes we search and search for something only to realize we already have everything we need. If we would open up our eyes to all the possibilities and the wonderful things that happen to us every day, I am positive that each and every day would be the best day ever. I used to think otherwise: I used to believe that there was only one person who could "complete" you. Now, many years later, I have come to the realization that my life is already fulfilling and full of love. Every day there is Joy waiting for me!

You don't have to be in a relationship to receive the benefits that love can provide. You just need to love yourself and have the love of friends. True friends inspire us, they support us, and make us feel better about ourselves. I am lucky to have friends all over the world. I have lived in many places, and along this jumbled path, I have made some amazing folks who have become lifelong friends. These friends have shown me real love, and shown me how to love. Love is bountiful. It should be part of your work-out plan to spend time with your best friends! The laughter alone is a workout and a calorie burner. So, fall in love with your friends and family again!

Thank you to my mother Catherine and my little sister Ada for helping me with the editing of this book. You help to mask my borderline illiteracy! Thank you to Bill Hoenk Photography for capturing the book photo. You make me look as good as I feel and I thank you for that. Thank you to my family and friends who have been so supportive of me and this venture. I couldn't have written this book, nor been so successful, without your love and support. Being loved for who you are makes life easy and worth living. A sincere heartfelt thank you to anyone who has ever inspired me, broken my heart, or made me laugh. I thank you for the experiences, good and bad.

In no particular order (and I apologize if I inadvertently omit anyone) thank you to: Catherine Flanagan Stover, John H. Stover, AdaRuth Stover, Perry Stover Wotring, Cora Stover, Ada Stover, Dorothy Locke, Jen Hanlon, Donna and Kevin Hanlon, Lynn and Frank Cushing, Ruth Ann Flanagan, Liz Flanagan, Dan and Janet Flanagan, Erin Flanagan Roberts, Reyna Kerzic, Kelly Miller, Catherine Tran, Julie Darby, Amanda Morgan, Janine Mauldin, Meri Lepore, Sabrina Clark, Kay, Jessica Handley, Don Wotring, Bill Hoenk, Eli Stover, Isaiah Stover, and Brett Morneau.

Quick Reference Guide

-Drink Wine

-Spoonful of Olive Oil when hungry, a spoonful in the morning and before you go to bed

-3 oz of Dark Chocolate

-Eat a couple of nuts before a meal

-Eat good fats like avocados

-Chia seeds - Two spoonfuls a day

-Eat lots of fruits and veggies especially pineapples, oranges, bananas and green veggies

-Drink Green Tea - 5 cups a day

-Say "I love you"

-Eat "clean" foods, nothing processed

-Skip the "junk" unless you make it yourself

-Enjoy sex with a partner, or by yourself.

-Laugh all day, everyday

-And, above all, LOVE!

About the Author

Dorothy Stover is a good girl with mischievous tendencies (nicknamed "Naughty-Dottie" at a very young age by her parental units.)

She has been in love with life for years now, and doesn't expect that to change any time soon.

She loves active-and-inactive-activities.

She listens to her Mother: "Intelligent people are never bored."

At times, Dorothy had a difficult relationship. With herself. But, making the decision to be a "victor" instead of a "victim" has allowed her to build a solid, healthy relationship. With herself. What has evolved is a committed relationship (with herself) constructed on a foundation of friendship, trust, excitement, hope, and always LOVE!

Follow her blog a www.lazypersonaltraining.com or find her on Twitter with the rest of the mainstream celebrities at @Doro727.

Sexercises:

I've heard this a 1000 times...sex is great exercise. More than likely you may already know most of these positions. I'm just trying to remind you of how much fun they can be and explain how they may tone your body. Bonus: I personally inked the stick figure drawings, your welcome.

Enjoy!

Missionary - Core and Buttocks

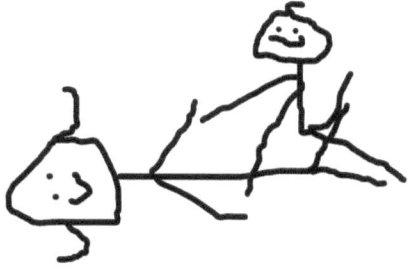

Missionary

In my opinion the missionary position is underrated. Often women think they don't have to do much besides just lie there. It can be some work being on the bottom. It can also be a lot of fun. In this position, the man is on top and the woman is on the bottom. When your partner thrusts towards you, the female should thrust back using her core and tighten her buttocks. Also, if you lift your pelvis up and hold this, this will be a variation on the missionary. Both will work your core muscles as well as your buttocks. Another variation is to do pelvic circles when he thrusts towards you.

Table - Everything

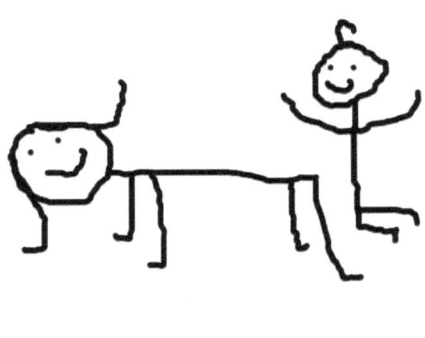

Table

This position is not the easiest but every muscle group will be engaged as you preform it. You will need some flexibility and some strength. Even doing this position for a 30 seconds will help to tone those muscles. For this position the female will move herself into a crab-like position with the male entering from the front. He should be on his knees. This will work all muscle groups to help stabilized, thrust and keep her balance.

Arch - Everything

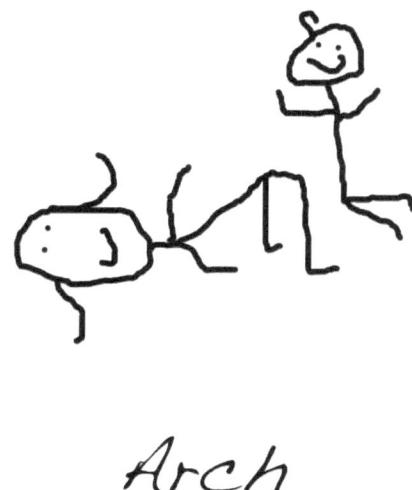

Arch

This is a variation on the Table position. The female will just lower her shoulders to the bed while keeping her pelvis up. She will use her arms, core and legs to keep her stabilized and to thrust. Do not tense up in the neck or shoulders. Take deep breathes and relax.

Lotus - Core and Glutes

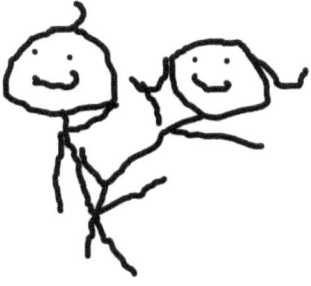

Lotus

This position always reminds me of the Karma Sutra. Not only for the name but also because you're wrapped up in each other. It's a very loving position with your bodies being very close and eye gazing galore. For this position the male is sitting up almost Indian style. The female will be on top straddling him. She will use her core and her glutes to thrust and keep her stable. A variation for the female is having one or both legs on his shoulders, this will then engage her arms since she will need them to keep herself stable, while using her core to thrust.

Scissors - Core and Inner-Thighs

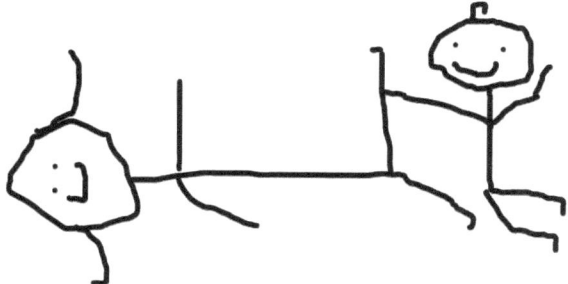

Scissors

This position allows for gentle and slow love making with deep penetration. The female should be lying down on her side with one leg in the air over her partner. She will be using her core and inner-thighs to keep herself stable.

Standing - Depending on the position: Arms, Core and Legs

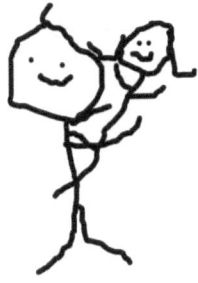

Standing

It's fun to get out of the bed and do something a little bit different. For this position, the male with have to hold the female.

This position has a few variations:

She may have both legs around his waist. She will use her upper body and core to keep herself stabilized as well as help to thrust.

Depending on height of each partner the male and female can be facing each other. The female will need to use her core and her legs to keep herself stabilized and to thrust.

The male would be holding one of the female's legs. Her core and leg muscles will work in unison to keep her balanced.

Feet around his neck. This position requires some flexibility from the female and strength from the male. The male will be holding the female and the female will have her legs up in the air and her feet wrapped around his neck. She will need to use her core and arms to keep herself stable. She may use her leg muscles to thrust.

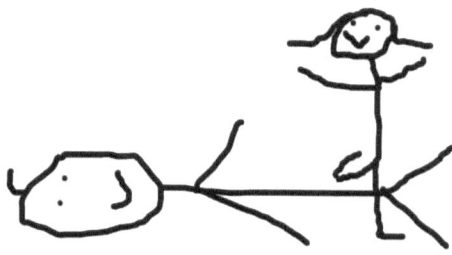

Cowgirl

CowGirl (Yee-Haw!) - Core and Buttocks

For this position, the female is on top of the male. The female should straddle the male, much like a cowgirl straddles a horse. The female will need her core and buttocks to keep her stable and to thrust.

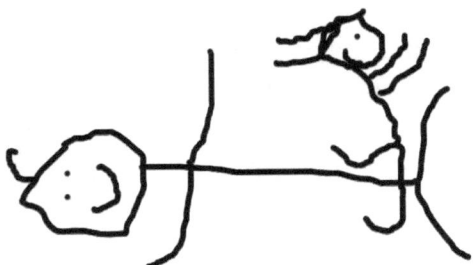

Reverse CowGirl

Reverse CowGirl

For this position, the female should straddle the male on top facing away from him. So it's the Cowgirl, just in reverse. Do you see where I'm going with this? This position works your core, as well as your butt. So not only will your partner love the view of your back, you'll also be toning your backside. It's a win win.

Semi-Split - Core, Legs and Butt

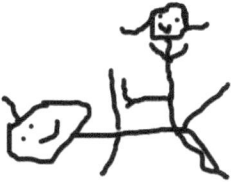

Split

This is a variation on the Cowgirl position. The female is on top of the male with one leg bent behind her and one leg bent in front of her. This should feel like a good stretch and the female will need her legs and core to keep her stabilized and to thrust.

1st Doggy Style Position - Core, Quadriceps and Glutes

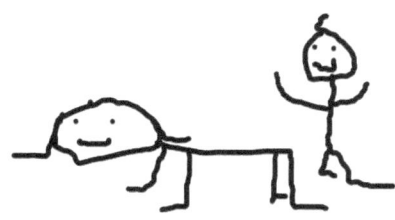

Doggie Style I

This position the man enters the female from behind. The female should be on all fours, with her hands flat on the ground or bed. The female should use her core to stabilize herself and her legs to thrust when the man thrusts. One variation on this for the female to raise one leg up in the air, like she were a dog about to pee. She will need to engage her core to stay stable. To get an even workout switch legs.

2nd Doggy Style Position - Core, Quadriceps, Glutes, Shoulders and Arms

Dogie Style II

This position the man enters the female from behind. The female should be kneeling with her hands up against the wall or on an object in front of her like a bed post. When the male thrusts, she will use her upper body to thrust back. One variation on this is for the female to do a circular motion with her hips. This will engage her core even more.

The Wheelbarrow - Core and Upper Body

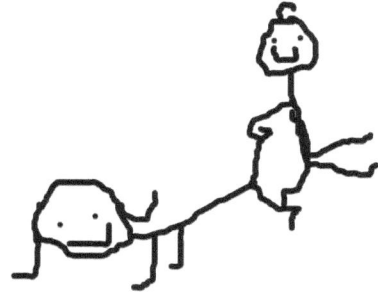

Wheelbarrow

For this position, first be in the doggy style position where the male is behind the female and she is on all fours. The male should hold both her legs up off the ground or bed. The female should tighten her core and engage her arms.

Dragon - Core and Arms

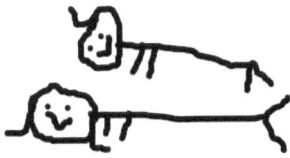

For this position, the female is lying face-down, her body straight. The male enters from behind directly on-top of her. She uses her core to thrust and she uses her arms to stabilize as well as stimulate the clitoris.